T0271700

SUN'S DANCE OF THE CHANNELS

Understanding Channel Interactions and Holography

JONATHAN SHUBS

Illustrated by Christina Malouf

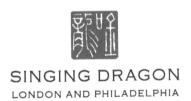

SINGING DRAGON
LONDON AND PHILADELPHIA

First published in Great Britain in 2023 by Singing
Dragon, an imprint of Jessica Kingsley Publishers
An Hachette Company

1

ISBN 978 1 83997 223 2
eISBN 978 1 83997 224 9

Printed and bound in the United States by Integrated Books International

Jessica Kingsley Publishers' policy is to use papers that are natural,
renewable, and recyclable products and made from wood grown in
sustainable forests. The logging and manufacturing processes are expected
to conform to the environmental regulations of the country of origin.

Jessica Kingsley Publishers
Carmelite House
50 Victoria Embankment
London EC4Y 0DZ

www.singingdragon.com

Sun's Dance of the Channels

by the same author

Sun's Season of Channels
An Introduction to Chinese Philosophy, Chinese
Medical Theory, and Channels
Jonathan Shubs
Illustrated by Fergus Byrne
ISBN 978 1 78775 902 2
eISBN 978 1 78775 903 9

of related interest

Essential Pulse Diagnosis
Mai Jing A-B-C Method
Jamie Hamilton Lic. Ac. LicCCHM
ISBN 978 1 83997 145 7
eISBN 978 1 83997 146 4

The Eight Extraordinary Vessels
Mikschal (Dolma) Johanison D.Ac., L.Ac.
Contributing Editor: Devon Gray L.Ac., MAOM, Dipl.OM
ISBN 978 1 78775 831 5
eISBN 978 1 78775 832 2

The Fundamentals of Acupuncture
Nigel Ching
Foreword by Charles Buck
ISBN 978 1 84819 313 0
eISBN 978 0 85701 266 1

The Art and Practice of Diagnosis in Chinese Medicine
Nigel Ching
ISBN 978 1 84819 314 7
eISBN 978 0 85701 267 8

CONTENTS

Part III: Systems of Channel Interactions

Space-Based Channel Interactions

Time-Based Channel Interactions

Exposure to Sunlight-Based Channel Interactions

Part IV: Putting it into Practice

Acknowledgements

It takes a community to raise a child…and write a book. There are so many people who either directly or indirectly have influenced, helped, and participated in this work, and I would like to name just a few to thank them.

First, I would like to thank my two mentors in Chinese medicine. Daniel Deriaz was my first teacher, and he not only shared his knowledge generously, but he also encouraged my own exploration and questioning of the material. The other main influence from a teaching point of view was the late Dr. Richard Tan. His work in synthesizing channel interactions into an accessible and clinically applicable system was a great gift to the acupuncture community. And on a personal note, I am truly grateful for his generosity and support of my work.

Second, I would like to thank all my patients, colleagues, and the participants of my courses. My patients, for their trust in allowing me to continue to refine and understand the clinical applications of theory. My colleagues at Chiway Academy, and especially Simon Becker, for their support and belief in the value of this material. And past participants of my courses—I learn more from them and their questioning than I can ever give to them.

Third, the individuals who were instrumental in the writing of this work. Christina Malouf, for her excellent images and precious collaboration. Hiba Samawi, for reading the early version and giving me feedback, support, and a better understanding of the psychological processes that the characters are going through. Bijan Doroudian and Anthony Monteith, for reading the early manuscript and giving me precious feedback from a practitioner's point of view. And finally, Claire Wilson and the whole Singing Dragon team, for their support and collaboration.

Finally, I would like to thank my family and friends, for putting up with me and teaching me about life. This is especially true for my two kids, Xavier and Adrien, who teach me more every day than I thought possible. Their mother, Elise Shubs, for raising our kids with me and supporting me in my professional career. And Denitsa Penova, for her support and encouragement.

INTRODUCTION

Thank you for taking the time to read this book. You may be a seasoned acupuncturist, a new practitioner, a student of Chinese medicine, a therapist in another domain, or someone who is just interested in how the channel system interacts. Regardless of where you are starting from, I hope you find value in this book. This book contains some technical talk and references that those without knowledge of Chinese medicine may find slightly more difficult to grasp. However, these parts can be skipped over without losing the value of the information.

I suggest that you read the book in the order that it was written. The book is written as a story featuring the characters of two older grandparents (Grandparents Terra) and their grandchild Sun. Sun visits their grandparents over the summer and learns about the channels over afternoon tea. The channel information is shared through the story, with each chapter building on the foundations laid before it in previous chapters. Once you have made your way through the book, feel free to go back and reread any chapter to better understand that aspect of the theory.

I would also like to share how this book came to be. The main theory explained in this book is what I call Unified Acupuncture Theory (UAT). This involves taking many different aspects of acupuncture, Chinese medicine, and channel theories and presenting a coherent approach to understanding how they all work. It is like the string that connects all the other theories that are out there, sort of like one theory to unify them all (and that is the name of the chapter that introduces the UAT model). I did not create the channel interactions that form the basis of the theory. That can be credited to Choo Chi Yin, who was the first person to present them in the 1970s, and Dr. Richard Tan, who taught them internationally for many years until he passed away in 2016. In fact, it was while I was sitting in a course with Dr. Tan that the theory was born. Dr. Tan would teach five of the six systems that I describe in this book. He would talk about the systems and give a theoretical explanation for each. For three of the systems, he would use the logic from the Ba Gua or eight trigrams that are from the *I Ching* (*Book of Changes*). For the other two systems, he used the logic from the channel clock. I was sitting in his course, mesmerized by the beauty of the systems and frustrated at not having one model to logically explain them all. That evening, I went to eat with other participants from the course and was talking about how I felt uneasy about the lack of a single theory. No one else shared my discomfort so I tried to let it go. But that evening when I was back in my hotel room I could not sleep. I stayed up till 4 in the morning thinking about and coming up with a logical, coherent, and complete theory that would explain all these interactions. And it was then that the UAT model was born. I will not bore you with all the thought process that went into it, but the next morning I went back to the course and showed my theory to Dr. Tan. He just looked at me and smiled. He said yes, that is it. He suggested I write an article to present my theory, which I did, and it was published in the *Journal of Chinese Medicine*.[1]

---

1   Shubs, J. (2012) 'The Foundations of Channel Theory.' *Journal of Chinese Medicine*, 100, 53–62.

That was over ten years ago. Since then, I have been teaching this theory along with more advanced applications of it internationally. And I finally felt that it was time to write it as a book.

First, though, I had to write the previous book, *Sun's Season of Channels*, also published by Singing Dragon, which lays the groundwork for the structure of the UAT model. This book is a continuation of *Sun's Season of Channels* and you are invited to read them together.

So that is the story of how and why I came to write this book. As I mentioned, this book is written as a story, with the main character being Sun. The gender, age, and nationality of Sun are completely ambiguous. This is done on purpose to allow the reader to choose whatever image they want of our hero—therefore, the gender-neutral pronoun of "they" is used for Sun.

Finally, a note to anyone who has attended courses by Dr. Tan or has studied his Balance Method. You will find many similarities in my UAT and his teachings. The differences that can be noticed are the explanations on the theory of why the channels interact and how to determine the nature of their interaction. In addition to the differences in the theory, the numbering of the channel interaction systems is different, and System 3 Closed Circuit Channels was not included in Dr. Tan's teaching—although many of his more advanced students named it System 7, it was never part of the official teaching. The table on the next page shows the correspondences between the UAT model and Dr. Tan's Balance Method.

With all that said, I hope that you will enjoy spending a summer with Sun and the Grandparents Terra!

UAT name	UAT system number	Dr. Tan's name	Dr. Tan's system number
Interior-Exterior	1	Internal-External Pairs	3
Full Channels	2	Chinese Channel Name Sharing	1
Closed Circuit Channels	3	NA	NA
Biorhythm Neighbors	4	Chinese Clock Neighbors	5
Biorhythm Opposites	5	Chinese Clock Opposites	4
Exposure to Sunlight	6	Branching Channels	2

PART I

HOLOGRAPHY, IMAGES, AND MIRRORING

CHAPTER 1

SUN ARRIVES TO VISIT THEIR GRANDPARENTS FOR THE SUMMER

The Idea of Local and Distal Uses of the Channels

The familiar sound of the metal on metal of the train wheels was becoming a rhythmic meditation for Sun. The bright yellow of the sun's rays streaking across the interior of the train, creating dancing light beams on the other passengers and the interior, was exposing images of the play of the world. Sun was in a trance, an almost meditative state where imagination and reality were talking with each other. Sun was contemplating everything that had happened since the last summer when they spent their holidays with their grandparents. They had discovered the basic concepts of Chinese medicine. The interplay of Yin and Yang, the cycles and interdependence of the five elements, the logic of the biorhythm clock, and, of course, the channels and how they are placed on the body. All this was conveyed to Sun by their wise and loving grandparents. A sense of gratitude and being at home swept over Sun as these thoughts entered their mind.

Sun was also thinking about this summer. When the

train comes to a stop, a new adventure would begin. Sun was returning to their grandparents for another summer. Expectations were high. They wanted to explore how the channels and the acupuncture points on them worked. They were sure their grandparents would share this information freely, and also give them other knowledge they hadn't even imagined yet.

The train came to a slow stop and Sun was awakened from their daydream. They gathered their belongings and got off the train. Waiting on the platform were Grandfather and Grandmother Terra, with patient smiles and a gleam in their eyes, full of joy seeing their grandchild one year older. They walked slowly toward each other, enjoying the moment and the eventual hug that was inevitable and much anticipated.

They walked to the car with big smiles on their faces, having been reunited after all these months. There was a little small talk. "How was the train journey?" asked Grandfather Terra. "Uneventful and calm," replied Sun. "We have prepared your room, just like last summer," explained Grandmother Terra. "Thank you," replied Sun. Although only these basic words were spoken, a much deeper communication was taking place. If words were put to it, Grandparents Terra would say, "We are happy to be together again and have missed you." And Sun would say, "I have missed you too and am ready for another adventure of the mind that only you can show me."

They got to the house and unpacked Sun's bags from the car. Sun went to their room and put everything away for the summer. The grandparents started to prepare the tea and they all met on the porch once everything was ready.

Teatime on the porch was their tradition. It was the time and place to talk about acupuncture and the universe. During the day, they would garden, go for walks, and just enjoy being with each other. At teatime, they would discuss, teach, learn, and share. For Sun, it was their favorite moments with their grandparents.

They all sat around the table as Grandfather Terra poured tea for each of them. Once the tea had been served and the first sip had warmed their mouth, Sun spoke with a smile, "So, let's get down to it. I have spent a whole year looking at the channels and reading books on the acupuncture points. And I have questions. Questions I think that you will be able to answer."

Both grandparents laughed. "We expected nothing less of you. And we are sure that your questions will be just as interesting as the answers we will try to give," said Grandmother Terra. "Where shall we begin?"

Sun answered, "I have been looking at the points and how they are described in the books. Locating them is easy now that I understand the placement of the channels from last summer. Where I am having difficulty now is understanding why the different points work. For example, there are points on the foot that say they treat headaches, or there are points that have indications that are so many that it seems like just using that point will treat the whole body. I know that the choice of points is a key principle in acupuncture, and it seems very confusing to me. Could we spend this summer understanding how the points work?"

Grandmother Terra smiled as she responded, "As usual, you have picked up on one of the most important and complex aspects of acupuncture. And yes, we will spend this summer looking at how we can understand and decide on the points. As you are aware, your grandfather and I have a different approach to understanding the aspects of Chinese medicine from that presented by the more traditional books. And this is also true for understanding the points. We respect and think the traditional form of giving actions and indications to points is important, but we will explain them more in relationship to systems and logic. This is the best way to start understanding them. It helps bring out the indications and actions of the points and makes them more accessible."

Grandfather Terra continued, "You have probably noticed that the indications can be put into two main categories. One category is that the point influences the area directly around where it is found on the body. For example, a point at the wrist will treat problems of the wrist. This is the easiest and most obvious use of the points. And we are sure you understand this without explanation." Sun nodded in agreement.

Grandfather Terra went on, "The points also have other indications or functions that take place away from where the acupoint is located. This is probably what you want us to explain."

Sun responded, "Yes, that's it. I could see that a point on the wrist will treat a problem on the wrist of the same channel. That much I got. It was the other uses that I had difficulty understanding. That is what I would like to know."

Grandmother Terra was happy to go on. "To understand the distal uses of the points we will have to revisit and expand some old theories and visit some new theories. So just like last summer when you wanted to know about where the channels were, and we went back to the beginning and looked at the theories that allowed us to understand the channels in a logical way. This summer we will do the same for the points. We will understand that points actions are based on a mix of what we can call the family of points and the holography of the body.

"The family of points means that a point can be associated with a group of other points that all share the same nature. This nature can be related to the five elements, the internal channels, or specific functions that the group has. The main families are:

- Five Element points

  - On each main channel, there will be a point that

is associated with one of the five elements. We studied these elements last summer. They are fire, earth, metal, water, and wood. These points will bring the quality of their associated element to the channel that they are placed on. So, for example, on the Foot Shao Yin Kidney channel there will be one point of each element. We know the Kidney is associated with the water element. This means that if we use the point associated with metal on the water element it will bring the metal energy into water and the Kidneys. This is the basis of what is called five element acupuncture.

- Yuan or Source points

  - This group of points is often grouped with the Five Element points and are given the name the Shu or transporting points. Each channel has one of these points. On the Yin channels, they are the same as the point that is associated with the earth point and on the Yang channels they are normally placed between the wood and the fire points. These points are used to remind the channel and the associated organ of their original function. There is a type of Qi called Yuan or Source Qi that is strong in these points.

- Luo or Connecting points

  - In each element there is a pairing of a Yin and Yang organ and channel, as well as many other associations. These associations include the sense organs in the face. These points are the communicators between the Yin-Yang pairs in the element and the sense organs in the head. For example, the metal element has the Hand Tai Yin channel, which is associated with the Lung, and the Hand Yang Ming channel, which is associated with the Large Intestine. These two channels together are also associated with the nose on the face. The connecting point on the Yin channel will connect with the Yang channel at the Source point. The connecting point of the Yang channel will connect with the face and the nose.

- Xi or Cleft points

  - These points are also known as emergency points. Each channel has one of these points and it helps the channel when it is in an emergency. That means when the channel really needs help.

"All these points are mainly located between the tips of the fingers and toes up to the elbows and knees. There are a few exceptions though.

"These families of points can help us understand some of the functions. However, we will not concentrate on them this summer. What we will look at is called the holography of points."

Sun had been following, and although they did not remember all the families, they could see the logic of them quite easily. But the last sentence was different. "What do you mean by holography of points?"

Grandfather Terra smiled. "Of course, this is a very different idea. The holography of points is about looking at where the point is and the channel it is on. Each placement will have links or connections to other parts in the body. We will study these links and understand their logic. Once we know which areas the point interacts with we will then look at the channels and see which channel the point can interact with. The holography of the points has two main theories:

one is the images that the area treats and the other is the interactions with the channel. This will be what we focus on this summer."

Sun said, "I think I get it but I am not quite sure. We are looking at the point as having two main pieces of information. The first is where it is on the body. The second is the channel interactions. And these two pieces of information together help us to understand its functions and actions. But I am not quite sure how this looks."

Grandfather Terra pointed to a place on his ankle. "First, we look at the structure that my finger is pointing to. In this case, it is my right ankle. Second, we identify the channel. In this case, it is the Foot Shao Yin Kidney channel. We will then look for a place that interacts with the ankle and at that place we will find a channel that interacts with the Foot Shao Yin Kidney channel."

Sun nodded. "If it is on the ankle, you will show me where the ankle can be connected to elsewhere on the body. And once I have found the area to treat, we will look at which channels will have an effect on that particular part of the ankle."

"You've got it, Sun." The grandparents beamed in unison.

Grandfather Terra said, "We will start tomorrow. I am getting hungry for dinner now."

CHAPTER 2

PATTERNS AND NATURE

Mathematical Basis of Holography

Sun woke with a sense of happiness and wellbeing. They loved waking up to the smells and sounds of their grandparents' home. It was a safe and comforting place where Sun was able to question the world and express themselves freely. This was a contrast for Sun from their day-to-day routine at school with their teachers and friends. Their grandparents challenged them and got Sun to think about things in a different way. At school, Sun felt limited by the teachers, not allowed to question and think about things. It felt like being brainwashed to think in a very limited way. And now they had weeks of respite from the limitations and felt free to be themselves.

Sun got out of bed and went downstairs to find their grandparents already up and making breakfast. A bowl of porridge was waiting for Sun, as well as two happy people full of cheer and joy.

Grandfather Terra smiled at Sun as they sat down at the table. "I do believe that you like fresh fruit on your porridge," he said as he cut a banana and some berries for them. "Today we thought we would go for a hike, to get you acquainted with the forest again. How does that sound to you?"

Sun took the fruit and put it on their porridge. "I would like that very much. After the train ride yesterday, I am feeling anxious and that will be good for me."

After breakfast, they set out with walking sticks and a packed picnic. They would stop and have lunch by the stream that led up to the mountains. Sun remembered this place well. Last summer it was where they discussed the five elements and how they interact. It was a happy place for Sun.

They walked for about two hours before stopping by the stream. Sun had not seen the time go by. They were enthralled by the smells of the flowers, the gentle rustle of the wind in the trees and grass, and the general buzz of life that surrounded them. It was a break from their normal life and they were happy. They stopped to set up the picnic. They took out sandwiches and fruit, and boiled some water to make tea. When Sun saw the tea come out, they knew that it would be OK to talk. And they were anxious to get to learning from their grandparents.

Once the tea was served, Sun looked at Grandmother Terra and said, "I am very happy to be here with you two. This is where I feel most alive and free. And also, where I can ask questions. I do not feel as if that is possible back home."

Grandmother Terra smiled and responded, "We are also happy that you feel good here. And we are aware of how you struggle at school. Perhaps we can talk about what is bothering you and try to help."

Sun looked at their grandmother and nodded. "It would be nice to have someone who understands me and what I am going through. But today I just want to be in this moment and start learning. We will have the whole summer to talk about it."

"OK," replied Grandfather Terra. "Where shall we start?"

"Well, I would like to know about how acupuncture works. Why, when you put a needle in one part of the body, it has an effect on a different part of the body."

Grandfather Terra nodded. "Of course that is what you want to know. Well, perhaps we should start with something a bit more global before we get into how it works. The first thing is to remember how Chinese medicine and acupuncture started. It started by observing nature and looking for patterns. You remember the five elements and how they were images of the world that were then used to explain how the body works?"

Sun replied, "Yes, I was thinking about that this morning while we were getting ready for this walk. This was the exact place where we talked about them last year. The five elements are:

- Fire

- Earth

- Metal

- Water

- Wood.

"Each element corresponds to a particular energy in the world as well as in the body. Yes, I remember."

Grandmother Terra smiled. "Good. That is exactly right. The five elements are about looking at patterns in nature and then using them on the human body. There are other patterns that we can observe in nature which we can then use to understand how acupuncture works. In the field of mathematics, the study of observation of patterns in nature is called mathematical biology. This was first started by a man named Alan Turing. You may have heard of him at school. He is credited with being the father of computing. He also looked at the patterns in nature and sought to understand them.

"The first step is to look at the outside world and identify patterns. These can be found in the stars and galaxies, in the waves of the ocean, and many other places. For example, snowflakes follow a pattern that can be observed. The observation of these patterns can then be seen in the human body. The two main patterns that we will use to understand how acupuncture works are the golden ratio and the Mandelbrot Theory, which includes the idea of fractals."

Sun looked slightly confused. "What does mathematics have to do with acupuncture? I am good at math at school, but I cannot see how it will help me understand how the points work."

Grandfather Terra smiled. "It is true that at first look they are not related. However, if you look closely at mathematics, you will find that it is a language to describe and understand the universe. In our modern age, mathematics is the tool that is used to explain the underlying principles of all material. It is used in chemistry, physics, biology, and most other scientific disciplines. We are showing how some of these principles can help us understand why Chinese medicine works and connect acupuncture to modern thinking. It is a way to bridge the gap between an ancient medicine and modern perceptions. It is also the language that most scientists use, so it makes sense to start here before we go into the more complex ideas."

"OK, I can accept that," replied Sun.

"So, as I was saying," continued Grandmother Terra, "there are two main ideas from the mathematical world we can look at. Let's start with what is called fractals. There is a whole field of research looking at this pattern. In its simplest form, it is saying that if we look at a whole object and zoom in on a section of the object, the pattern will be the same."

Sun had a questioning look on their face.

Grandfather Terra intervened. "Take a look at that tree. You can see the trunk, which then has branches coming off it. And those branches have other branches coming off them. Now, if we look at the whole tree, we see a tree. If we just look at one branch and its smaller branches, we see the same pattern. This is an example of a fractal."

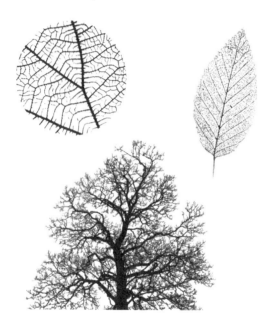

Sun nodded. "I see. It is as if the branch is a smaller tree. Can you give me another example?"

"Of course," said Grandfather Terra. "Think about rivers and streams. Small streams feed into rivers and rivers feed into bigger rivers and this continues until they get to the sea or the ocean. And when we look it has the same branching pattern as a tree. Also, we can look at snowflakes. They follow the same pattern. Or even lightning. Electricity uses fractals all the time when it is not constrained by wires. We also find it in plants and how they grow their leaves.

"Now, how about the human body? Can you think of any examples of fractals in the human body?"

Sun nodded. "I remember studying the lungs in class and thinking how they looked like trees. They have branches that get smaller and smaller. Also, the cardiovascular system. All the arteries and veins have the same image."

"Excellent," replied Grandmother Terra. "The lungs and the cardiovascular system are great examples. We could add the brain and the nervous system. All these systems contain fractals.

"So that is the first mathematical concept we will use. The second is the golden ratio, which has many names. Sometimes it is referred as the golden proportion or Phi, and is the basis of a series of numbers called the Fibonacci sequence. Have you ever heard of this?"

Sun shook their head. "I don't think so."

Grandfather Terra explained, "The golden ratio is about proportions. It describes how two segments of something relate to each other in an optimal way. It is saying that the smaller segment is in the same proportion to the bigger as the bigger segment is to the two segments together. I know that sounds like a lot of words, but I will try to show you." He picked up a branch lying on the ground. "Here we have a stick. I can divide the stick into two parts. We see that both sides have the same length. This is the perfect balance point, and the ratio is one to one. This means that each segment is the same length. Now, the golden ratio does not use this idea. If I move the separation of the two segments off the center I would find that I would have a golden ratio. Here, the small segment is in relationship to the big segment. And the big segment is in the same relationship to the whole stick. Look at your thumb. The smaller more distal bone compared to the bigger bone has roughly the same ratio as the big bone to the whole thumb. This ratio is said to be 1.618. It is often shown like this:

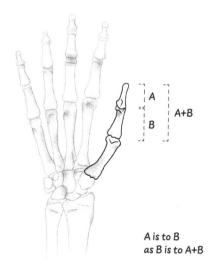

A is to B
as B is to A+B

"This relationship between A to B and A + B is called Phi or uses the symbol from the Greek letter Φ.

"There is also a sequence of numbers that use this ratio. It is 1, 1, 2, 3, 5, 8, 13, 21, 34... This is called the Fibonacci sequence.

"This Phi or golden ratio is often combined with the idea of fractals to describe how the fractals are made. When we were talking about the tree before, we saw that the whole tree looked like the branch with the smaller branches. Well, the pattern where the smaller stems branch out uses Phi. They branch out at the point where the golden ratio is."

Sun was able to follow but was not sure they understood everything. "So, in nature we find fractals. That is, a part of something resembles the whole of it. And there is a pattern to how things branch or divide. And the golden ratio, which has lots of math involved to explain it, is the pattern the fractals use. We find this in the outside world, like trees, snowflakes, rivers, and things like that, and also in the human body. In the human body, you gave me examples of the respiratory system, the cardiovascular system, the nervous system, and the brain.

"So, this is an example of how math finds patterns in nature and compares them to the human body. This seems very far from Chinese medicine. And did they even have this mathematics back then?"

Laughing, Grandfather Terra responded, "We do not have any reference to the ancient Chinese being aware of the Fibonacci sequence. However, we find that these ideas have been part of both Eastern and Western culture for centuries if not millennia. The golden ratio is used in art very often. Leonardo Da Vinci drew the Vitruvian Man in about 1490. This drawing shows the proportions of the human body, and it follows the golden ratio. In ancient India, we find geometric patterns that are fractals and use the golden ratio over and over again. So, we can see that although we can only recently talk about them in mathematical language, this observation of the world has been present for a very long time. And this helps to understand how the imaging and mirroring which we will talk about soon works."

"OK," said Sun. "I guess I shouldn't have expected you to give me the simple answer right away. You always build up to it using all these extra ideas. I guess you two will never change on this point!"

The grandparents were laughing. Grandmother Terra said, "Yes, Sun. We like to take things from the beginning and build them up. So, thank you for indulging us and now we can finish our picnic and start heading back. We wouldn't want to miss our afternoon tea on the porch."

CHAPTER 3

AN ARM FOR AN ARM AND A LEG FOR A LEG

Holography and Mirroring

The hike back was full of peace and wonder. Sun was looking at the world around them with new eyes. They were seeing patterns in almost everything they looked at. And seeing all these patterns was starting to open up an idea of the human body that they had not realized before. They could hardly wait until they could ask more questions, and knew that letting the questions bubble inside would make the answers much more interesting. They were starting to remember that patience could be a good thing. They had no time for it at school but here it almost seemed like the only path to take.

Once the trio had returned and unpacked from the hike, they went to the porch for their afternoon tea.

Sun poured the tea and started talking. "These summers with you two are really special to me, and I feel comfortable with you. I find your way of explaining things and sharing with me motivates me to want to know more. I have been thinking this year. Every time I meet an adult, they ask me what I want to be when I grow up. Sometimes I respond by saying that I want to still be me but older, or that I do not know. And now I feel that I will say that I want to be an acupuncturist like my grandparents."

Both grandparents smiled in unison. Grandfather Terra took a sip of his tea and looked lovingly at Sun with a mixture of pride and a little sadness. "We would be very proud to see you become an acupuncturist, Sun. And we will willingly share with you all our experience. But at the same time, I think your first answer is the best one. There is no need to know what you want to do in the future. You are still young and have so much yet to experience. The question asked by adults is more about them than you. And this might be part of your difficulty at school. Do you remember when you were very little, after your first year of school, what you said to us?"

Sun shook their head. "I said lots of things to you. Could you be more precise?"

"You said that you were afraid that school would take your imagination and creativity away from you. Do you remember that?"

"To be honest, not really. But it does sound like how I felt, and still feel."

"Our response to you was that no one can take away your creativity and imagination. Those are yours for ever. Some people will try, but if you want to hold on to them, they will always be there for you. You were right in sensing that there was a danger for this to happen. A lot of people feel as if they have to let go of a part of who they are to fit in to society. And they expect others to do the same. When you are asked questions like that, often it is about people wanting confirmation that they made the correct choice in letting a part of them be suppressed to succeed. Your answer about staying the same person just older is a brilliant one."

Grandmother Terra raised her cup at Sun. "We are proud of who you have become as a person and who you are still becoming. It would be our honor to teach you more about acupuncture, Sun."

Sun blushed a bit and felt very happy inside. They were amazed that their grandparents remembered them thinking about their creativity when they were little. And then to avoid becoming too mushy Sun said, "Well, are you going to teach me or not? How do the patterns we saw this morning relate to acupuncture?"

Everyone laughed. "Very well, Sun," responded Grandmother Terra. "Let's put the patterns to work. The first thing we will look at is holography. Holography is about seeing how different parts of the body interact. The more similar they are, the more effect they can have on each other. So, we will look at which parts of the body are similar and how they connect to each other.

"The easiest place to start is with the arms and the legs. Do you know how many bones there are in the arms?"

"I guess I could count them, but I am sure you can just tell me."

"There are 30 bones in the arm and hand:

One bone in the upper arm

Two bones in the forearm

Eight bones in the wrist

Five bones in the hand

Fourteen finger bones.

"And how about the leg and foot?"

"Well, knowing you, there are probably 30 bones there too."

"Very smart, Sun. Yes, there are 30 bones in the leg and the foot:

One in the upper thigh

One at the knee

Two in the lower leg

Seven in the ankle

Five in the foot

Fourteen in the toes.

"So, we have very similar structures between the arms and legs and the hands and feet. We can also see this in the joints or articulations. They have similar structures and ranges of movements. Putting this all together, we can mirror the arm on to the leg, and vice versa."

Sun got the gist but asked, "What do you mean by mirroring?"

Grandfather Terra responded, "By mirroring, we mean that we can make associations between these two limbs. And we use the word mirror because they are like mirror images of each other. We will see later on that we use a different word for the rest of the body.

"So, let's take a look at this picture of the arms and the legs next to each other.

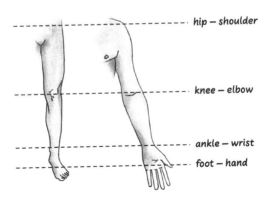

Normal Mirror of the Arm to Leg

"Here we see that the shoulder and the hip are mirrors of each other, the elbow and the knee are mirrors of each other, the wrist and the ankle are mirrors of each other, and the hand and the foot are mirrors of each other. So, if the problem is on the shoulder, I can look for a place on the hip to interact with it."

Sun looked at the image and said, "So, if the shoulder interacts with the hip, then it will also be true for the other pairs. So the elbow will treat the knee, the wrist will treat the ankle, and the hand will treat the foot. And that is also true in the other sense. The hip will interact with the shoulder, the knee with the elbow, the ankle with the wrist, and the foot with the hand. But what if the problem is between the shoulder and the elbow?"

"A very good question," replied Grandmother Terra. "We would look for a similar place between the hip and the knee. The key is to think in proportions. If the problem is one third distal to the shoulder and two thirds proximal from the elbow, then we would look for a place that is one third distal from the hip and two thirds proximal from the knee."

"OK," said Sun. "I think I get it. We look for similar areas on the leg to treat the arm and on the arm to treat the leg."

Grandfather Terra nodded. "That's it, Sun. That is what we call the normal mirror because the arms and the legs line up almost perfectly. Now let's take the idea of the golden ratio we saw earlier today. Remember how there was one segment that was longer than the other segment and they had a relationship between them and the whole? Well, the arms and legs fit that pattern."

Sun smiled. "I was thinking about this earlier. I was thinking about how the arms seem to have this golden ratio between the upper arm which is longer and the forearm which is shorter. I wasn't sure if they met the golden ratio though."

"Well, they are close. Nothing is exact but they are close enough for us to use it. As this ratio creates a strong connection to nature, we can also use it for mirroring. This time we will mirror the smaller segment to the larger segment of the opposite limb. It looks like this image."

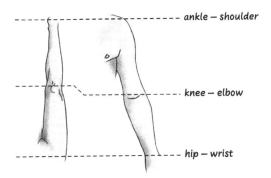

ankle – shoulder

knee – elbow

hip – wrist

Reversed Mirror of the Arm and Leg

Sun looked at the image and thought. "OK. So here one of the limbs is flipped and then they are put next to each other. If I am seeing this right, here the shoulder and the ankle interact, the elbow and the knee interact, and finally the wrist and the hip interact. And does the part between the shoulder and the elbow also interact with the part between the knee and the hip?"

Grandmother Terra nodded. "Yes it does. That's it, Sun. If we have a problem at the shoulder, we can look for points around the hips or the ankles. And if the problem is distal to the shoulder, then we look for points distal to the hip or proximal to the ankle."

Sun looked contemplative. Finally, they said, "What about the other shoulder? If there is a problem with the left shoulder, can I use the right shoulder? Or even the right wrist? And what about left and right in the opposite limb? With the shoulder problem, can I use either hip and either ankle?"

Grandmother Terra responded, "Let's try to answer one question at a time. The arms can also treat the arms. And as you said, we can use the normal mirror or what we call the reverse mirror. So, for example, the right shoulder can interact with the left shoulder and the left wrist:

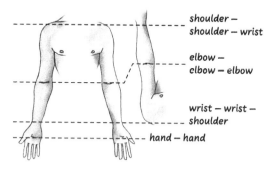

shoulder –
shoulder – wrist

elbow –
elbow – elbow

wrist – wrist –
shoulder

hand – hand

Both Reversed and Normal Mirror of the Arm to Arm

"And the same is true for the legs. The right hip can interact with the left hip and the left ankle:

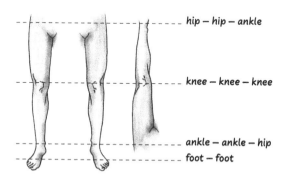

hip – hip – ankle

knee – knee – knee

ankle – ankle – hip
foot – foot

Both Reversed and Normal Mirror of the Leg to Leg

"Now when we are going from arm to arm or leg to leg, we are always going to the opposite side. If we weren't we would be treating locally, and that is not what we are looking at here. However, when it comes to the arm interacting with the leg or vice versa, the idea of left and right will depend on the channel that we choose. We will look at that later. For the moment, we are just understanding the mirroring."

Sun said, "OK, let me see if I've got the whole picture. The arms with the hands and the legs with the feet mirror each other. This is because they have very similar structures. By mirroring we mean that they interact or treat each other. We can use the joints to guide us. So, the shoulder mirrors the hip, the elbow the knee, the wrist the ankle, and the hand the foot. If the problem is between two articulations, we look for areas that are also between the two corresponding articulations. That is the normal mirror.

"There is also the reversed mirror which uses the golden ratio. Here the shoulder mirrors the ankle, the elbow still to the knee, and the wrist to the hip. The idea between these areas uses the same principle as before.

"And finally, the arm can treat the other arm both as a normal mirror and a reversed mirror. This is also true for the legs."

Grandfather Terra was grinning with pride. "You are as bright as ever, Sun."

And they got ready for dinner.

CHAPTER 4

AS ABOVE, SO BELOW

Holography of the Limbs to the Body

Sun was woken by Grandfather Terra knocking on their door asking if they would like to do some Qi Gong. Sun got out of bed to join in with pleasure. These were the movements that their grandparents did every day and which they said were part of why they were so healthy. The three went to the field behind the house and started following a series of movements that the grandparents called the The Crane Form of Qi Life Qi Gong. As they explained the form to Sun, they told them to imagine they were imitating a crane and that all the movements were the different actions a crane would do, such as spreading the wings, flying, hunting for food, and swimming in water. Remembering the ideas of patterns from the day before, Sun not only noticed the flow to the movements but also the many connections between the different parts of their body.

The arms and legs were like counterweights, each helping the other to make the movement more precise. And Sun also felt connections in their body. When they were able to relax their wrists, their neck felt different. They also felt a sense of wellbeing and calm in their body as they did more actions.

It was a very interesting experience. Sun decided to practice with their grandparents every morning.

After a day of gardening, having lunch, and going for a walk, they were all ready for afternoon tea. Grandfather Terra brought out the tea set and started the little ceremony they had built up. First, tea was served, and everyone took the time to taste the flavor and savor it. Only after that first sip had been fully experienced did they begin talking. This time, the grandparents were ready for Sun's need to learn before Sun could even ask.

Grandfather Terra began, "So, yesterday we looked at how there were patterns in nature that we can use to understand the human body. And we saw how the arms and the legs are mirrors of each other and how they can be used to treat each other. Today we will look at how the arms and legs can be used to treat the whole body."

Sun smiled. "I was thinking about that. This morning while we were doing our Qi Gong, I noticed that the sensations I was feeling in my body were often started by moving one of my arms or legs. I felt that when we did the exercise with the wrist, I could feel my neck relax. Is this one of the associations?"

Grandmother Terra nodded. "Yes Sun, that is one of the associations and we will get there soon enough. First, let's give these types of associations a name. Yesterday, we used the word mirroring for mapping the arms to the legs and vice versa. Today, we will map the limbs to the torso and the head. As the structures are not as clear as they are with the limbs, we will have to use our imagination a little bit more, so we will call this imaging. We will take the references we saw yesterday on the limbs and transpose or map them onto the rest of the body.

"So, the first image we will look at is one where we use the whole limbs with the hands and the feet and put them with the torso and the head. Do you remember the puppet show we took you to a few years back?"

Sun smiled. "Yes. It was a silly story about a princess who fell in love with a prince because he had saved her. I enjoyed it at the time but now find it not very believable. Just because the prince saved her, does that really mean that they would be happy together? They hardly knew each other, and they were supposed to live happily ever after. My parents took a long time to get to know each other before they were married, and they still aren't always happy with each other. But I am sure that is not what you are asking."

Grandfather Terra was laughing. "That is the show Sun. And yes, the story does seem far-fetched, but we were asking if you remembered the puppeteers that we met after the show, and how they let you try the puppets. Afterwards you were walking around using your hand to speak as if it was a head. And of course, the stories you came up with were much better than the show."

Sun smiled. "Yes, I remember. You two indulged me until it was dinnertime and then told me I couldn't feed my hand but let me eat with my hands. Well, we were eating burgers."

Grandmother Terra replied, "Exactly. You were using your hand as the head of the puppet and the body was over your arm. Well, that is the first image we will use. The hand will be the head and the arm will be the body. And as we saw yesterday, the hand can also be the foot and the arm the leg. So, we will see that the head is the hand and foot, and the body is the arm and leg."

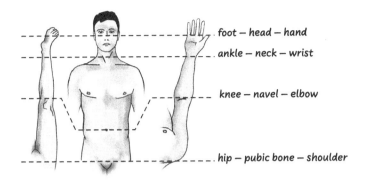

foot – head – hand

ankle – neck – wrist

knee – navel – elbow

hip – pubic bone – shoulder

Normal Image of Limbs to Whole Body

Sun looked at the image and started to explain what they saw. "So, the head is the hand and foot. The neck is the wrist and ankle, the navel is the forearm and lower leg, and the pubic bone is the shoulder and hip. This would explain the relation between my wrists and the neck from this morning."

Grandfather Terra replied, "That is correct. In the points books, you will find that there are many points that are in the hand and the feet that are indicated for problems in the head. Some of the examples are Hegu LI 4, Xaingu ST 43, Houxi SI 3, Shugu BL 65, and Taichong LIV 3. All these points are either in the hand or foot and treat problems that are in the head. Once we understand that the hands and feet are images of the head, we can better understand the indications of these points. And we can do the same for the rest of the images.

"Using this image, we associate the elbow and knee with the navel. This means that if there is pain or discomfort at this horizontal level of the body, we can use points at the middle joint of the limbs. This makes me think of one point in particular. The point at the elbow on the Hand Yang Ming Large Intestine channel is called Quchi LI 11. This point is indicated for many digestive problems. There is another point on the Foot Yang Ming Stomach channel that is called

Zusanli ST 36, and this point has many of the same indications. The difference between these two points is that Zusanli ST 36 is located distal to the knee, whereas Quchi LI 11 is located at the elbow. So when the problem is at the navel line, Quchi LI 11 will work better, and when the problem is above the navel line, Zusanli ST 36 will work better as it is distal to the knee which images above the navel. This is an important distinction that is often not talked about in the books. They give a general indication of the area that the point treats, but do not talk about the image, so both will have indications for abdominal pain, but they treat different areas of the abdomen. And using the imaging we can make a better choice."

Sun followed for the most part. "Grandfather Terra is going into professor mode!" Sun said with a smirk. "I do not remember all the points as I haven't studied all of acupuncture that much, but I see what you are saying. The images help explain which area the points will treat. I imagine that this will also need the channels to make the full picture."

Grandmother Terra laughed. "Yes, Grandfather Terra has that tendency when he gets excited. And you are correct that imaging will tell us the horizontal area that the point will treat, and then we use the channels and how they interact to see which vertical segment it will interact with. We use both pieces of information together. However, for the moment we are only looking at the images and will get to the channel interactions later.

"So, we have the main correspondences:

Head—Hand—Foot

Neck—Wrist—Ankle

Navel—Elbow—Knee

Pubic bone—Shoulder—Hip.

"And the areas in between use the proportion to map the torso and the limbs. So, a problem in the chest will be closer to the wrist and ankle and further from the elbow and knee, as the upper chest is closer to the neck and further from the navel."

Sun nodded. "I get it. Just like yesterday. We use the main references of the joints on the legs and certain anatomical structures on the torso to make the connections. If a problem is between these references, we map the problem onto the limb using the same proportions between the references. Is there also a reversed image of this?"

Grandfather Terra chimed in, "Yes, I do go into professor mode sometimes. And yes, there is a reversed image. However, it is slightly different as we will leave out the hands and feet. It looks like this image."

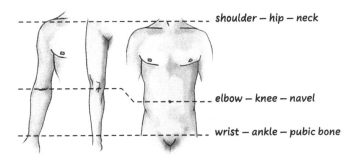

shoulder – hip – neck

elbow – knee – navel

wrist – ankle – pubic bone

Reverse Image of Limbs to Body without the Head

Sun looked at the new image. "Oh, I see. Here the elbow and the knee are still linked to the navel, but the other joints have changed their position. So, the hip and the shoulder are now linked to the neck and the ankle, and the wrist is linked to the pubic bone. So, the point you said that was distal to the knee before, Zusanli ST 36, will now treat below the navel. It treats above and below the navel but not the navel itself. For that I need the other point."

Grandfather Terra nodded. "Yes, that is it. The other point was Quchi LI 11, and it only treats the navel here as it is at the elbow. So, just like for the mirroring, in the images we also have the reversed and normal images.

"And now we will show you the last main image that we can use. That is of the whole head to the limbs. We already saw that we can use the hands and the feet to image the head. Sometimes we need to be more precise, and the hands and the feet can be quite small to get a perfect image. So, we blow up the image of the head and map it onto the limbs."

Grandmother Terra showed another two images.

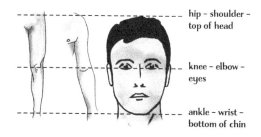

Normal Image of Limbs to Whole Head

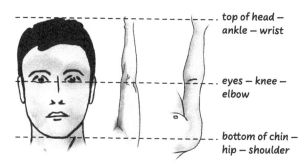

Reverse Image of Limbs to Whole Head

Sun studied the images carefully and took a moment to reflect. After a few moments, they looked up at the grandparents and started to say what they thought. "So, the limbs can also image the head. The shoulders and hips are either the top of the head or the bottom of the head depending on whether the image is reversed or not. The same is true for the wrist and the ankle. And the elbows and the knees are always the eyes in either image. So, if I were to take the main parts of the face, I would have the following images I could use:

Part of the head	Arm		Leg	
	Normal image	Reversed image	Normal image	Reversed image
Sides of the head	Middle of upper arm	Middle of forearm	Middle of thigh	Middle of lower leg
Forehead	Middle of upper arm	Middle of forearm	Middle of thigh	Middle of lower leg
Eyes	Elbow	Elbow	Knee	Knee
Ears	Just below the elbow	Just above the elbow	Just below the knee	Just above the knee
Cheeks	Just below the elbow	Just above the elbow	Just below the knee	Just above the knee
Nose	Middle of forearm	Middle of upper arm	Middle of lower leg	Middle of thigh
Mouth	One fourth away from wrist	One fourth away from shoulder	One fourth away from ankle	One fourth away from hip

"In fact, it is all proportional, just like the rest of the images."

Both grandparents were nodding and smiling. "As always, it is a pleasure to teach you, Sun," replied Grandmother Terra. "You have understood the idea of imaging and mirroring and how to think with proportion in the images."

Sun smiled and then continued to look at the images as the tea went cold and they decided to call it a day there.

CHAPTER 5

LIKE TREATS LIKE, IMAGE TREATS IMAGE

Micro Systems and Other Forms of Holography

Sun was up and awake before the grandparents and was waiting for them in the field ready for Qi Gong. Following the movements of their grandparents, Sun felt like a bird soaring high above looking down on the world and completely free, and then they felt as they imagined a tree must feel, with roots going down into the earth and absorbing the energy of the world through their feet. It was indeed a wonderful feeling and they felt refreshed and calm at the end of the series.

The day went like all the other days. Breakfast, gardening, lunch, a walk, and finally teatime. Although Sun still saw teatime as the highlight of the day, they also were starting to appreciate the routine and the time when they were not learning about acupuncture. They noticed that they would find themselves daydreaming and seeing images everywhere. And their grandparents would engage in the images with them, asking them not just to describe what they saw but to also create stories with them. This was not like it was at school, where they had to explain their creativity—here they were allowed to live it. They would spend the whole morning talking about the flower and the journey it went through from bud to bloom. At moments, Sun felt the flower and was the flower, and at other moments, they were the soil that held the roots in place; they could also be the nectar that the bee was taking. All the while, Sun was still Sun, and they were more than themselves. Sun thought how simple it was to be themselves and how perhaps they could hold on to this knowing.

Teatime came and Sun was ready for the next lesson. Once the tea was served and they all had taken that first sip to savor and connect to the tea, they started to talk.

Grandfather Terra began, "So, Sun, before we move on from the images, do you have any questions?"

Sun responded, "Of course I do. Are those the only images? If not, how many other kinds of images are there? And why are we only looking at using distal images? Can we also just put the needle where the problem is?"

"All good questions and we will try to answer them. Let's start with the last question first. Why do we use images and distal points? Well, there are many systems of acupuncture that do use local points for both pain treatments and internal functional problems. And these systems can work very well. They include what are called trigger points, motor points, or, in Chinese, Achi points, and they all have their uses. We are focusing on the distal treatments for a few reasons.

"First, when it comes to pain, if the patient has discomfort at a certain place, we don't want to increase the pain at that place. Also, if we put a needle in a wrist that is in pain, we cannot then ask the patient to move the wrist to see how the pain has changed. When we use a distal point, for example in the ankle, the patient can then move the wrist to see how the affected area is responding to the treatment.

"Second, when we put a needle at the location of the problem, only the area around the problem is being called to action. By using distal treatments, we are including all of the body. The information has to travel through different channels and different parts of the body, and each of those parts is then included in the treatment. This ties in to the idea of a holistic approach where we do not treat the symptom but we treat the person with the symptom.

"Third, we are using the logic and application of distal points to understand why the distal points work. It is not saying that local points do not work or have their place. However, studying the images and the channel interactions, we can understand the use of distal points and choose the best point or points for the patient."

Sun nodded. "OK, I get that. So distal points and images are not the only way to do acupuncture, but by studying them and using them we can understand the concepts of acupuncture better and also interact with the patient in different ways."

Grandmother Terra nodded. "Yes, Sun, that is true. And Grandfather Terra left out one factor that we both think is important. *Like treats like* or *image treats image*. This means that when we are inserting a needle into a point on a channel, there is a story behind the point that interacts with a story in the person. The idea of the channels that we spent last summer learning is in fact just a story—one that speaks to the story in the patient. And the images we are using speak to the images in the patient.

"When we were talking about the puppet show, you said how the story did not talk to you or, we could say, it did not resonate with you. And because of this you did not hold on to the story and forgot it until we reminded you of it. This is the same idea. If the image we use does not resonate with the patient, then the patient will not be receptive to the information that is in the story. And this is an important component in the patient getting better. The patient's body must be able to understand what is being said to it through the needles. And as the body is part of nature, we can use the images in nature to talk to the patient. This is true of the five elements, the channels, and the images we have seen these last two days."

Sun felt as if they understood and did not understand at the same time. "I think I can see a bit of what you are saying and yet I do not fully understand it. *Like treats like, image treats image.* This sort of makes sense. Is it saying that there has to be a connection between the two, a bridge of some sort? And how similar does the bridge have to be for it to work?"

Nodding, Grandfather Terra responded, "It is not an exact science but a moving and living dynamic. Just like Yin and Yang. Something that we see as Yin can only be perceived in relationship to something that is Yang, and vice versa. And, the image of Yin is also in Yang as they both are looking somewhere but from different viewpoints. The way images work is the same. They have a commonality that is shared and yet they are different. If there is no commonality, then they cannot interact with each other, and if there is no change of perspective, then they cannot react to each other. We will see this relationship requirement when we look at channel interactions too, as they are also a sort of image of each other."

Sun nodded. "OK, I see that. And what about my other questions?"

Grandmother Terra laughed. "Always ready for the next bit. OK. You also asked whether there are different images. And I think you know the answer will be yes. We can classify the other images into two different groups. Images that work with the channel interactions and images that don't. For the images that use the channel interactions, there are many. In fact, the number is only limited by your imagination. We can take any part of the human body and map it onto another part. The key is to keep the proportions the same.

"Of these types of images there are three main ones.

From a system called Master Tung Acupuncture, they are called the large, medium, and small Taiji:

The large Taiji uses the fingers to the elbow or the toes to the knee to map the rest of the body. The elbow and the knee are one limit of the image, and the tips of the toes and fingers are another end of the image.

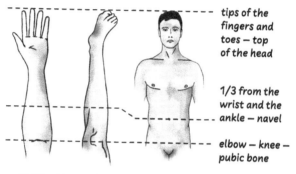

tips of the fingers and toes — top of the head

1/3 from the wrist and the ankle — navel

elbow — knee — pubic bone

Large Taiji — Normal Image of Limbs to Whole Head and Body

The medium Taiji uses the fingers to the middle of the forearm or the toes to the middle of the lower leg to map the rest of the body.

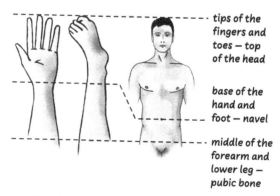

tips of the fingers and toes — top of the head

base of the hand and foot — navel

middle of the forearm and lower leg — pubic bone

Medium Taiji — Normal Image of Limbs to Whole Head and Body

And the small Taiji uses any bone to map to the rest. The most common is the 2nd metacarpal bone. This is the bone in the hand that connects to the index finger.

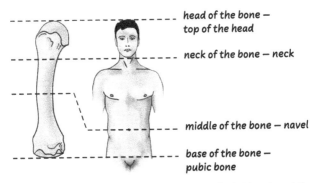

head of the bone – top of the head

neck of the bone – neck

middle of the bone – navel

base of the bone – pubic bone

Small Taiji – Normal Image of Limbs to Whole Head and Body

"Of course, each of these images can be mapped onto other limbs, just the head, or just the body. And they can also be inversed as we did with the images yesterday."

Sun looked at these images and saw that they were not that different than the ones they saw days before. "So, in these images the key is to define the limits of the images and then map them out. Any part can image another part of the body as long as the proportions are used correctly."

Grandfather Terra agreed. "In these types of images, the key is matching the proportions. Now, with the images that don't need the channel interactions it is slightly different. And there are many styles of acupuncture and other healing modalities that are based on them. These are full systems in themselves, and we will just name a few of them but not go into details of how they work here:

Abdominal acupuncture: uses an image from the *I Ching* on the abdomen to treat the whole body.

Auricular acupuncture: uses an image of the whole body in the ear.

Hand acupuncture: uses the whole image of the body on the hand.

Foot reflexology: uses the whole image of the body on the sole of the foot.

"And there are many others—too many to mention. But I think you get the point."

Sun agreed. "Yes, I see that there are many more systems of acupuncture than I could have imagined, and they must all have their uses. And also, for once, I would like to thank you for not making it more complicated by explaining all these different systems. I will have enough time to learn them once I have understood the basics I think."

"It is very wise of you, Sun, to not ask for too much information," replied Grandmother Terra. "And on that note, let's get ready for dinner."

PART II

UNDERSTANDING THE BASIC THEORY

CHAPTER 6

STARTING AT THE BEGINNING

The Theory for Channel Interactions

Sun felt disconcerted the following day. On the previous day, they had felt alive and part of the world. Yet, on this day, things seemed dimmer, darker, as if they were missing some light. This disturbed Sun doubly: first because of the dimness and second because of the contradiction to the previous day. How could they go from being so alive to feeling like this in a short time when nothing had really changed? Sun decided it was time to talk to their grandparents about this as it was something that happened often during the year.

As they were going for a walk, Sun started to open up to them. "I do not understand. Yesterday I felt like the sun, bright and full of energy. Today I feel like the soil, dark and not wanting to move. I cannot identify what has changed from yesterday to today, yet something in me has changed. And I feel like this often. What is going on?"

Grandfather Terra stopped, walked slowly to Sun, put down his backpack, and took off Sun's. Then he took Sun in his arms and just held them there. At first, Sun resisted, not wanting to let anyone touch them and not feeling like being hugged. Grandfather Terra started to release the hug when he felt Sun's resistance, but as he released, Sun started to hug him back and wouldn't let go. So, Grandfather Terra held them in his arms and just was there. Tears started to form in Sun's eyes and their breathing became shallow. Sun started to cry and could not stop. Grandfather Terra just held them with patience and empathy. Nothing was said and nothing was needed to be said. After a moment that was unidentifiable in time, Sun came back to themselves and let go of their grandfather.

Sun looked up and saw Grandmother Terra sitting there with some tea in a thermos. She handed a cup to Sun and told them to drink. The grandparents both just sat down close to Sun and were present for them. As Sun came back to themselves, they looked at their grandparents and started to smile. They still felt like they did before but a bit lighter and freer. "What is happening?" Sun asked.

Grandmother Terra replied, "You being human, that is what is happening. You are a complex person who has many emotions and feelings and they all have their place: the heavy, sticky, uncomfortable feelings, and the light, airy, joyful feelings. If we do not take time to acknowledge them and give them their space, they will overtake us at times. This moment was a moment for heavy feelings, and other moments are for other feelings. Who knows what the next moment will be like?"

"But I do not understand something. When I am at school, I am always expected to be happy and OK. All the other kids seem happy and OK. Yet I have these days of darkness and it makes me feel even worse that I do not see any other kids feel the same."

Grandfather Terra nodded. "That is often how it feels. When you are happy, the whole world is happy with you. When you are sad, you are sad alone. This might feel true and in some ways it is, but in reality, when you are sad or heavy, you are closer to yourself than at any other time. The spontaneous difficult emotions that we cannot place are whispers of your soul. The happy joyful moments are often the laughing of your spirit, and when we can laugh and cry together, we are uniting our spirit and soul. So today will be a soulful day. We can rejoice in it and allow it to be."

Grandmother Terra leaned forward and looked Sun in the eyes. "We all have days like this. And they are important to honor and cherish. All the people at school have days like this too, they just don't allow themselves to show it. Only the brave can allow it to come up and out. And you, Sun, are very brave indeed."

Sun finished the tea and sat in silence for a while feeling what they felt and pondering what had been said. They felt a strange lightness in their chest. Not a lightness of joy, but a lightness of sadness and sorrow moving. It was like a heaviness that did not change weight yet was more comfortable to hold. And at that moment, the image of Yin and Yang come back to their minds. The ever-changing dynamic that had been with their minds since last summer but had always been with their body.

Sun looked at their grandparents and smiled while shaking their head. "It seems that when I am with you two, everything makes sense. Even my difficult moments are easier here. Thank you. Now, to stop thinking about all this soul and spirit stuff, can we talk about how the channels interact?"

Grandfather Terra smiled warmly. "We are happy that we can be a place of comfort for you, Sun. And of course, let's start talking about the channels again. And to do that let's do a quick reminder of Yin and Yang and the five elements. This is how we understand which channels can interact with each other."

"OK. So, like with everything, you always want to start at the beginning."

Grandmother Terra commented, "It is always good to start with the beginning. And when it comes to channels, it is Yin and Yang. Do you remember the way we represented Yin and Yang using the lines?"

"Yes. We used a solid line for Yang and a broken line for Yin."

"Correct. And do you remember how they had different levels?"

"Yes. They went from the first level where Yin and Yang are separate, to the second level where there were variations of Yin and Yang, and then to the third level where there were eight variations. This was from the *I Ching* if I remember correctly."

Yin-Yang according to the I Ching

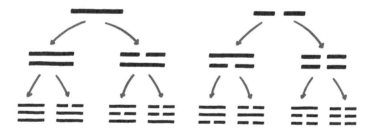

"That is correct, Sun. Excellent. And do you remember the five elements?"

"Yes, of course. They were:

- Fire

- Earth

- Metal

- Water

- Wood.

"And they each had a Yin channel and a Yang channel associated with them. They were also associated with the different lines of the *I Ching*, if I remember correctly."

"That is true. Each element has an association with one of the aspects of Yin and Yang, with channels, and many other associations that we looked at last year. To understand how the channels interact, we have a theory that uses these aspects: the Yin-Yang representation, the element, and the channels. Let's start with the associations of the Yin-Yang representations. As we saw, there is the top-down image that you were showed earlier. We can also organize the first two levels in a circular way that allows us to understand the cycles of Yin and Yang such as a day or a year, where we see how the sun and the absence of sun progress."

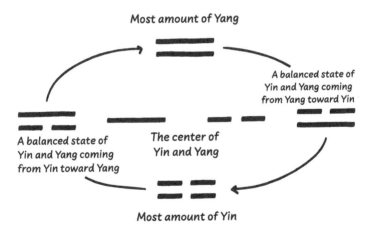

Most amount of Yang

A balanced state of Yin and Yang coming from Yang toward Yin

A balanced state of Yin and Yang coming from Yin toward Yang

The center of Yin and Yang

Most amount of Yin

Sun looked at the image and nodded. "Yes I remember this. We could add the seasons to this cycle. It looked like this:

Yin-Yang with the seasons

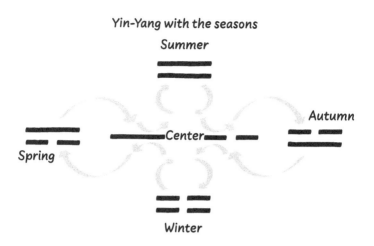

"And then we could put the elements instead of the seasons."

Yin-Yang with the five elements

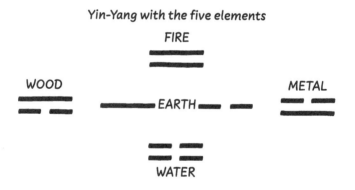

"That is perfect, Sun," replied Grandfather Terra. "You have remembered it all from last year. You have indeed been studying this summer. Now, I am getting hungry and would like to return for lunch. We can discuss more this afternoon during teatime."

Sun nodded and felt much better after talking about how they felt.

CHAPTER 7

THE SEPARATION OF HEAVEN AND EARTH

Including Heaven in the Five Elements

Sun still felt the heaviness for the rest of the day, but the heaviness felt lighter to carry. It was as if, just by talking about it, there was support to carry it. And that led Sun to another thought. Does the heaviness have to be carried or is there another way to honor it where it is not so heavy?

The ritual of preparing and sitting down for tea had been completed, so Sun started by revisiting what had happened earlier.

"I have been thinking about what you said earlier today and how we have to carry our heavy emotions sometimes. Is there another way other than just carrying them? It seems as if this will take a lot of energy."

Grandfather Terra responded, "Yes, there are other ways to interact with the heavy emotions. Most people will try to ignore them and put them in a place where they cannot be found. Or they will wallow in them and let them consume them. Both of these approaches are not really very healthy for the person. So, what can we do when we have the heavy emotions? Well, the first thing is to recognize that they are there and allow them to be there. All our emotions are important and need to be seen. This does not mean that we need to get stuck in them, but we do need to first allow them to be present. This is a first step. Next, we can start to work and interact with the emotion. And to do this it is helpful to see emotions as a response to something. The emotion is attempting to bring our attention to some aspect of ourselves. We could even say that every emotion has a function. It is there to help us identify what is happening. In Chinese medical thought we concentrate on five main emotions, and they can be linked to the five elements. We would say that each element has one primary emotion associated with it:

Water is associated with fear

Wood is associated with anger

Fire is associated with joy

Metal is associated with sadness

Earth is associated with thinking.

"All of these emotions are healthy and important to be felt as each has a function in dealing with life. Let's see if you can figure out the functions of the emotions."

Sun nodded. "That is a difficult idea. I have never thought of my emotions as having a function. I have always thought they were just something that I feel. And also, how is thinking an emotion? That seems a bit strange to me. I will try to imagine the functions though. Water is associated with fear, so what is the use of fear? I am not sure I see it."

Grandmother Terra agreed. "It is a different way of thinking about our emotions and, yes, thinking seems strange to be considered an emotion when we think about our emotions. We will come to thinking last. Let's start with water and fear. What types of situations do you feel fear in?"

"Let me see. I felt afraid when I was feeling very down earlier today. I was scared that I would always feel like that."

"OK, that is a good start. Could we rephrase that to say you felt there was a danger of you always feeling like that?"

"Yes. That is fair. There was danger in the air. So, are you telling me that fear is associated with the presence of danger?"

"That is exactly it. When we feel fear, a part of us is telling us that there is some danger. Now this danger can be physical, say we are up high and there is a possibility of falling, or there is a menacing energy, and we could get hurt. The fear can also be something inside that feels threatened. For example, the heaviness you felt this morning. That can feel as if it is threatening you not physically but psychologically or emotionally."

"I see. So, when I feel fear, it is a warning sign that there is some danger I need to be aware of. OK, what about anger then? I get angry with lots of people for so many different reasons that I do not see what the function could be."

Grandfather Terra responded this time. "Sun, when I first took you in my arms this morning and you resisted, how did you feel at that moment?"

"I was angry at you. I wanted to push you away. It felt as if you were breaking through something that I didn't want you to break through at first."

"That is the function of anger. It is to protect you. Your first reaction was to try to push me away because you were protecting yourself from all the other emotions. And if you think about when you get angry at people, most of the time it is because you feel they are invading some aspect of you. So, anger is about protecting your boundaries. Your boundaries are what give you a sense of who you are, and what's OK and not OK for you. So, anger is about preserving your integrity, either physically or psychologically."

"Yes, that makes sense. I was protecting myself from

the sadness I did not want to feel. So, what is the function of sadness then?"

"Sadness is about letting go. The emotion is telling us that there was something that we had that we no longer have, or something that we no longer need to hold on to. This is why when someone dies, the main emotion is sadness. It is informing us of the process of letting that person's physical presence go. It can be more complicated than just letting go but that is the essence of the function of sadness."

"OK. So, the three difficult emotions you mentioned (fear, anger, and sadness) are all like signs that I need to do or respond to something. How about joy? What function can joy have?"

"Think about when you feel joy. What are the situations that you feel joy in?"

"I feel joy when I am doing Qi Gong or talking with you two. I feel joy when I am playing or singing or doing something creative. And I feel joy when I am learning something interesting."

"And if you look at all these situations, you are experiencing joy when you are connected to something. You can be connected to us, to the creative endeavor, the interesting material you are learning, and so on. Joy is about connection. It is helping you connect to something important at that moment. So now we have talked about the main emotions except thinking, which we will do in a moment. But we can already see that emotions are signs that we need to respond to something. So, when we feel our heavy emotions, we can ask ourselves what emotion we are feeling and what its function might be. If we are feeling fear, then we can ask what the danger is. We can examine what is happening and identify where there might be something we feel is menacing. We can then address the situation itself and not stay just in the experience of feeling the fear. It is the same with anger. When you feel anger, ask yourself, what am

I protecting myself from? Do I really need to protect myself, and if so, what is the best way to respond to the threat? With sadness, we can ask ourselves what we are letting go of. Once we know this, we can then start the process of letting it go. And finally, with joy, we can do the same thing. When we feel joy, we can ask if we are connecting with something we want to connect with. And if so, do we continue to connect with it?"

"I think I understand. The emotion is telling me that I need to focus my attention on something and figure out what it is saying and how to respond to it."

Grandmother Terra smiled. "That is correct, Sun. And that brings us to thinking. Thinking is at the center of all the emotions. Once we feel the emotion, we then need to process the information that it is giving us and decide on a response. And this is why it is associated with the earth element. The earth is in the center of all the other elements, and thinking is in the center of all the other emotions. It is what allows us to process and understand the emotion. It also helps us to respond to the emotion. So, to answer your earlier question about how to work with your emotions instead of just carrying them or hiding them, we can see here that we have a path forward. First, we feel the emotion, then we identify the emotion, we then figure out what the emotion is pointing to, and finally we decide how to respond to the emotion. And we may need to do this many times to get through all the emotions we are experiencing."

"OK, I get it. So, the emotions are really only signals that I need to understand."

"Yes, that is exactly it. And there is a bit more than just understanding—there is also responding to them. This is a good moment to explain a bit of theory about the five elements that will help us understand channel interactions. You remember that we had five elements and twelve channels? And that it was difficult to understand how they fit together?"

"Yes, of course. The Pericardium and the Triple Warmer were the extra pair of organs and channels."

Grandfather Terra continued, "Yes, they are the two extra channels. Now if we combine the five elements and the images of the Yin-Yang lines, we will see this:

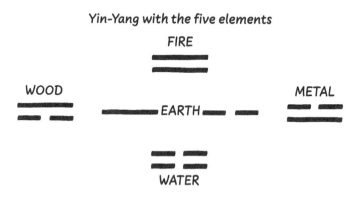

"And we see that the earth has both a Yin and a Yang line. And if we think about Yin and Yang, we can also say that it is the separation of heaven and earth. So, what we are suggesting is that in fact heaven is another element that is very close to earth. So, we could show the same image as:

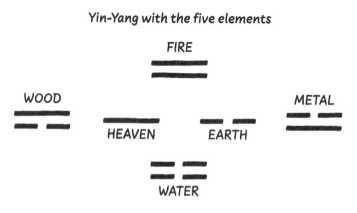

"Here we have both heaven and earth in the center. This means that they work together as a Yin-Yang pair. And if we assign the Pericardium and Triple Warmer to heaven, then we have a model that can incorporate all of the channels, organs, and elements together. We will look at this model tomorrow and see exactly how it works. But if we think about the emotions again, we can see how they all work together."

Sun spoke, "Hold on. You just added an element into a thousand-year-old system and you haven't mentioned it before?"

Grandmother Terra laughed. "Yes, Sun. Your grandfather and I have found that this model of adding heaven makes more logical sense to us and helps us understand a whole range of different things in Chinese medicine. We have developed our whole system of acupuncture on this concept of heaven being a sixth element that is closely related to earth. It is our invention, although there are many hints that it was in the older texts and then removed. But we will not bore you with these academic problems. This is a model that works for understanding how the channels interact as well as the emotions and many other aspects of the theory. Would you like us to show how this goes back to the emotions we were talking about?"

"Of course I would."

"Well. We have already said that the emotions are associated with the elements. We have:

Water associated with fear

Wood associated with anger

Fire associated with joy

Metal associated with sadness

Earth associated with thinking.

"And now we will add:

Heaven associated with creativity.

"We have the four outer emotions that are signals from the body that there is a response needed. Fear, anger, joy, and sadness are signaling the type of situation you are in and then the earth (thinking) needs to digest it. If you remember, the organs associated with earth are the spleen and stomach, which are all about digestion. Once it has been digested, a response may be needed, and this response needs some creativity. This is where heaven comes in. It allows us to be creative and imaginative with how we respond to the world. We could say the earth supports us and heaven inspires us."

Sun nodded. "I think I see it. There are the four main emotions that are signaling that we need to act in some way. They send the signal to the earth where they are digested and analyzed. Then a response is needed, and for that response to be complete it needs some creativity or imagination that comes from heaven. And heaven is the new element that is the counter to earth and is Yang in nature, where earth is Yin in nature. So, heaven and earth are a pair, just like Yin and Yang, and they are at the center of all the other emotions and elements."

"That's it, Sun! That is excellent! What is interesting is that we can use this system to help us understand and respond to our difficult emotions. And we will also use this heaven and earth pair to look at what we call the Unified Acupuncture Theory model tomorrow."

"OK. Sounds good to me."

CHAPTER 8

ONE THEORY TO UNIFY THEM ALL

The Unified Acupuncture Theory Model

The day started like all the other days. The routine of Qi Gong, breakfast, walking, gardening, lunch, more walking, and more gardening had helped Sun find balance and be more centered after yesterday's rollercoaster of emotions and explanations. Sun felt a little stronger now that they had more tools to work with their emotions and the knowledge that the emotions are just trying to tell them something. Emotions were no longer these big heavy things that couldn't be worked with. Sun was also really excited about the new theory that the grandparents had alluded to: the Unified Acupuncture Theory. What a grandiose title! And to think that they had developed it made Sun proud of being their grandchild, without even knowing what it was or if it worked. Something in Sun made them feel as if this theory was a big deal, and they were ready to learn about it.

Teatime came as usual and all three got ready on the porch with their tea, books, and love of knowledge. Tea was served and Sun could not hold off any longer.

"First, I want to thank you for yesterday and the teaching

and caring you shared with me. I felt stronger today and I think I might be stronger the next time I get flooded with all the emotions. I know it will still be difficult, and yet I feel as if I can handle it better.

"Now yesterday you talked about your Unified Acupuncture Theory. The name is quite big, and it reminds me of the search in physics for the Unified Field Theory or the Theory of Everything. Are you ready to share your secret with me?"

Both grandparents were smiling at Sun and laughing a little. They loved how Sun could be grateful, respectful, and rebellious all in the same breath.

Grandfather Terra responded, "Of course we will show you our humble secret theory. Except that it is not secret and the real key to it you already heard yesterday. The separation of the earth element into earth and heaven is the main point. Once we have this, we have six elements:

Metal

Water

Wood

Fire

Earth

Heaven.

"With six elements and six Yin channels and six Yang channels we have a model that is based on the number six. So let's start looking at it."

Grandmother Terra took out a drawing and showed it to Sun.

Yin-Yang with the five elements

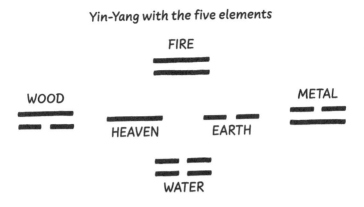

"Yesterday we finished with this image. We placed each of the elements plus heaven with one of the expressions of Yin and Yang. So here we have the classic cross pattern of the elements that can be used to describe the directions and seasons:

North, winter—water

East, spring—wood

South, summer—fire

West, autumn—metal

Center below, inter-season from wood to summer and summer to autumn—earth

Center above, inter-season from metal to winter and winter to summer—heaven.

"This cross pattern is very useful for describing these kinds of cyclical patterns and static positions. However, it is limited when describing movements and influences between the elements. So just like we did with the five elements last year, putting them in a different layout, we will do so with this image."

Sun said, "Yes, I remember that we put the five elements in a circular pattern where earth was between fire and metal. Will we use a circular pattern here?"

"Not quite. We will use a different system that will still have a center but is structured differently. First, we will look at the Yin-Yang lines and make three groups. Each group will have what we call balance between the elements. So the three groups are:

Wood and metal

Fire and water

Heaven and earth.

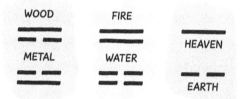

"We call these balanced because the Yin and Yang lines interact with each other. If there is a bottom Yin line in one element, there will be a bottom Yang line in the other element. And the same is true for the top lines. If one is Yang, the other will be Yin. Or if there is only one line, as in heaven and earth, they will be one Yin and one Yang line.

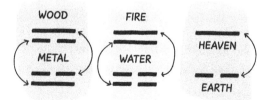

"Understanding these three pairs is the first step."

Sun looked at the images. "Yes, I see it. Wood and metal balance each other. They both have one Yin and one Yang line, but they are in opposite places in the element. So, the bottom line of metal, which is Yang, balances the bottom line of wood, which is Yin. And it is the opposite for the top lines. Metal has a Yin top line and wood and a Yang top line.

"Fire and water are a little different. Water is two Yin lines and fire is two Yang lines. So, the bottom lines together create a Yin-Yang pair, as do the top lines. And for heaven and earth, there is only one line. Heaven is Yang and earth is Yin, so they balance each other."

Grandfather Terra smiled. "Perfect, Sun, that is the idea. Once we have these three pairs, we can now rearrange them into a model. We will first describe the placements of the elements and then we will talk about the logic and how it applies to channels."

Sun nodded. "OK. Let's do it."

"We will start by putting the heaven and earth pair in the middle. This is because everything starts from the separation of heaven and earth. We will put heaven on the left side and earth on the right side.

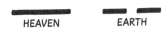

"Now we will put the fire and water pair on the earth side of the diagram.

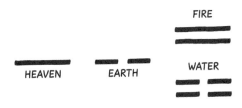

"And then we will put the wood and metal pair on the heaven side.

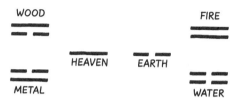

"So here we see that the three pairs are still in relationship with each other, except that heaven and earth are in a horizontal orientation and the wood metal and fire water are in a vertical orientation."

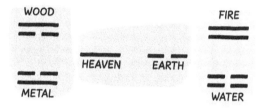

Sun looked at the images and understood the arrangement. "OK, I see that this is how you place these elements. Could you now tell me why and, more importantly, how they relate to the channels?"

Grandmother Terra nodded. "Of course. The first thing to notice is that the balance of the original pairs is preserved. Now the most common question is, why is the fire and water pair on the earth side and the wood and metal on the heaven side? Is this arbitrary or not? Of course, it is not arbitrary. To understand this, we use the nature of Yin and Yang to see it. Yang is said to control Yin, and Yin to nourish Yang. Yang is more volatile, whereas Yin is more stable. Heaven is more Yang, whereas earth is more Yin.

"Now if you look at the other two pairs, wood and metal not only balance each other but have balance in the element itself. Metal has a Yang bottom line and a Yin top line. Wood has the opposite, a Yin bottom line and a Yang top line. This means that the element has an equilibrium to it. Also, metal is associated with the autumn equinox when there is an equal amount of both day and night, and wood is associated with the spring equinox.

"The other pair of fire and water do have a balance between them. However, in their own elements they are extremes. Either Yang for fire or Yin for water. They represent the solstices which are extremes of day and night.

"So, wood and metal together and individually are more balanced and stable. Fire and water are balanced together but not individually. Fire and water need the stabilizing energy of the earth to help keep them balanced. And metal and wood need the movement energy of heaven to keep things moving."

Sun said, "OK. That makes sense. It is like fire and water are extremes so the earth can hold them and use its Yin energy to maintain some balance. Wood and metal are stable so need the heaven and Yang energy to help them move."

Grandfather Terra smiled. "Yes. So now that we understand the placement of the elements, let's bring in the channels and place them in the elements. We will do this in a logical way, starting by going back to the associations of the Yin and Yang organs. Do you remember these associations?"

Sun sat up straight, took on the air of the serious student, and began, "There are two main categories of organs. There are Yin organs and Yang organs. The Yin organs are the Kidneys, Liver, Spleen, Heart, Lungs, and Pericardium. The Yang organs are the Bladder, Gall Bladder, Stomach, Large Intestine, Small Intestine, and the Triple Warmer or Triple Heater. The Yin organs are more associated with the storing of Qi and its different functions, and the Yang organs are more about extracting the Qi from food and getting rid of the waste. We can associate each Yin organ with a Yang organ to make a Yin-Yang pair.

"If we look at the Yin organs, we see that there are three that are below the diaphragm and three that are above. The three that are below the diaphragm have a physical connection to one of the Yang organs. The Kidneys connect to the Bladder; the Liver connects to the Gall Bladder; and the Spleen, which also includes the pancreas, connects to the Stomach.

"The other three Yin organs create an image of the intestines. The Heart is at the center of the chest like the Small Intestine is in the center of the lower abdomen. The Lungs surround the Heart like the Large Intestine surrounds the Small Intestine. And the Pericardium is a membrane around the Heart and that is an image of the Triple Burner which might be the Mesentery.

"I remembered all this from last summer. And it is finally becoming useful. So, the associations are:

Kidneys with Bladder

Liver with Gall Bladder

Stomach with Spleen

Heart with Small Intestine

Lungs with Large Intestine

Pericardium with Triple Burner."

Sun was beaming at their grandparents. And they smiled and were lost somewhere between pride and laughter.

"Very good," said Grandmother Terra, in as serious a way as she could. "So, we have the pairs of organs that we know are also associated with channels in the body. We spent last summer talking about the placement of the channels, so we won't go over them now. We also know that the organs which are associated with channels are also associated with the elements. So, we will now put the organ/channel pairs on the model with the elements.

"If the physical Yin organ is below the diaphragm, it will be placed on an element that has a Yin line on the bottom; if the Yin organ is above the diaphragm, it will be placed on an element with a Yang line on the bottom. The Yang organ/channel will follow the Yin organ/channel.

"The elements with a lower Yin line are wood, water, and earth, so the channels associated with them are:

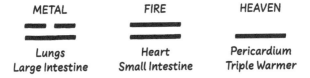

WOOD	WATER	EARTH
Liver	Kidneys	Spleen
Gall Bladder	Bladder	Stomach

"And the elements with a lower Yang line are metal, fire, and heaven, so the channels associated with them are:

METAL	FIRE	HEAVEN
Lungs	Heart	Pericardium
Large Intestine	Small Intestine	Triple Warmer

"The only new thing from last year here is that the Pericardium and Triple Burner are associated with heaven instead of fire. We talked about this yesterday. So now if we put it all together with the six elemental positions, the channels, and the organs, we get this diagram:

Unified Acupuncture Theory

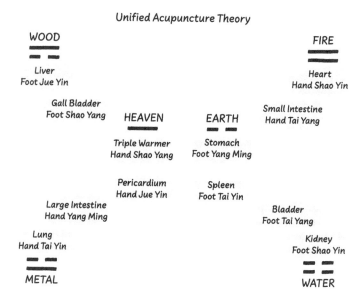

WOOD

Liver
Foot Jue Yin

Gall Bladder
Foot Shao Yang

HEAVEN

Triple Warmer
Hand Shao Yang

Pericardium
Hand Jue Yin

Large Intestine
Hand Yang Ming

Lung
Hand Tai Yin

METAL

FIRE

Heart
Hand Shao Yin

Small Intestine
Hand Tai Yang

EARTH

Stomach
Foot Yang Ming

Spleen
Foot Tai Yin

Bladder
Foot Tai Yang

Kidney
Foot Shao Yin

WATER

"This the Unified Acupuncture Theory model."

Sun looked at the image and then at their grandparents. "So you have created a new element so to speak called heaven, you have arranged the elements in a different manner where there is balance between the Yin and Yang lines, you have associated the channels with the elements based on the Yin organ placement, and you have placed the Pericardium and Triple Burner with heaven and not in fire as all the classics do, and you put them all into this image, which is very pretty and feels balanced. And then you tell me that this will explain how all the channels interact? OK, I guess I will believe you two." Sun could barely hold back the laughter as they were saying these words.

Grandfather Terra couldn't hold back his laughter. "Very fair, Sun. We have spent the whole time explaining this model and now you are wondering how it will help to understand the channel interactions. Well, that will have to wait for tomorrow as the tea is cold now."

CHAPTER 9

SAME, SAME BUT DIFFERENT

Rules for How Channels Can Interact

Sun had a lot to think about over the next day. The theories that the grandparents had shown them had made sense and Sun could see how they simplified some of the logic that was confusing from the previous summer—especially the introduction of heaven as a counter to earth and being associated with the Pericardium and Triple Burner. The fact that these two channels were no longer associated with fire made the whole channel system and five elements much more symmetrical and logical in Sun's mind. Sun was anxious to now learn about how this change would help to understand the channel interactions themselves. Well, they would have to wait for teatime.

And teatime came quite quickly. The day had passed by, and before Sun was aware of it they were already sitting on the porch and ready for the next lesson.

Sun looked at both grandparents and smiled. "I have been thinking about your Unified Acupuncture Theory and can see how it makes sense. However, I do not see quite how it will explain the channel interactions."

Grandfather Terra nodded. "Yes, Sun. We agree that it makes a lot of sense, and it clears up the complicated logic of the Pericardium and Triple Burner. As to the channel interactions, we will use the model to map out the interactions between the various channels. We will see that the placements of the channels arranged this way helps us better understand why these interactions work and some of the qualities of each interaction. The UAT model will be the basis for this."

"OK. Let's start then."

Grandmother Terra smiled. "Well, there is still one important thing to address before we start using the model. We need to come up with some rules for how the channels will interact. Everything needs rules to understand how it will work. And the UAT model with channel interactions is no different."

Sun shook their head. "Of course there are rules. What would the world be like without rules? Rules are everywhere. Fine. Let's look at the rules then."

Everyone was laughing. Grandmother Terra began, "So, to the rules. There are two parts to the rules. The first we will group as the similarity rule and the second as the polarity rule."

Sun was intrigued. "Similarity and polarity?"

"Yes Sun," replied Grandfather Terra. "Similarity and polarity. The similarity rule states that when two channels interact, they must have a similarity between them. There are three different types of similarities that channels can have:

Space

Time

Exposure to sunlight.

"Each time channels interact they must share one of these connections."

"What do you mean by space, time, and exposure to sunlight?"

"Well, when we are talking about space, we mean that the channels have to occupy the same special area of the body. When we were learning about the channels, we were able to categorize them into:

Front

Middle

Back.

"If the channels are sharing a space relationship, then they will both need to be in the same area of the body. So front channels will interact with other front channels, middle channels will interact with other middle channels, and back channels will interact with other back channels."

"Alright. So, there are some relationships that are based on space and this means that the channels occupy the same space on the body. So, for example, a front arm channel can interact with the other front hand channel or the foot front channels. Is that the idea?"

Grandmother Terra beamed. "Yes, that is exactly it. We will look at the space relationships in more detail later, but you've got the idea. We will see that there are three channel interaction systems that are based on space.

"The second type of similarity is time. Do you remember the channel clock?"

Sun rolled their eyes. "Of course I remember it. It was one of the most interesting parts of the theory we talked about last summer."

"Well, we use the channel clock to explain the time relationships. We have two relationships that are based on where the channels are situated on the clock. We use the name biorhythm to talk about the clock."

"So, space and time. There are three systems based on space and two based on time," said Sun.

"Yes, and there is one last relationship that is based on sunlight."

"What do you mean sunlight?"

Grandfather Terra chuckled. "When we look at the names of the channels we know that the name is referring to the amount of sunlight that each channel gets. For example, the word Tai means great, so the Foot Tai Yang means the channels on the foot that get the most or greatest amount of sun on the Yang side of the foot. The channels Arm Tai Yin also get the most amount of sun but on the Yin arm. So, these two channels are able to interact: the Foot Tai Yang and the Hand Tai Yin. This is what we mean about sunlight. Channels that get the same amount of sun respectively have an interaction."

Sun understood. "So, if I've got this right, there are six different types of channel interactions or six systems:

- Three based on *space*

- Two based on *time*

- One based on *sun*.

"And we're going to look at each system individually."

Grandmother Terra said, "Yes. That is perfect. There are six systems, and they are categorized exactly as you said. Now there is the second part of the interactions. This is what we call polarities. For anything to interact it must have on one hand a similarity and on the other something to contrast it to. This contrasting element we call polarities.

"Think about a conversation with someone. You need to have some basic similarities otherwise you won't be able to understand each other. There must be something that connects you. And you also need to have some differences. If you both agree on everything there is no real interaction.

There needs to be something that you differ on for it to become a conversation. Without the differences, it would be a short talk where you just agree with each other."

"I think I see. I remember someone explaining romantic relationships by saying that opposites attract. And when I asked them, they said that each person had to have some basic things they felt connected to in the other person and also things that were different about the other person for there to be a real attraction. Is this the same idea?"

"Yes. If two people don't agree on anything, they won't be able to connect. And at the same time, if they agree about everything, they will get bored of each other very fast. This is why we need some polarity in relationships, to keep things moving and interesting.

"When we talk about channels, we have three different polarities that we can observe:

Hand channels and foot channels

Yin channels and Yang channels

Channels on the right side of the body and channels on the left side of the body.

"The hand and foot channels we have already talked about. There are some channels that either stop or start at the fingers and cover the upper limbs; these are the arm channels. Their opposite are the channels that either stop or finish in the toes and cover the lower limbs; these are foot channels. When a foot channel interacts with a hand channel, this is a polarity."

"OK. Feet and hands are opposites, and when the channels interact, they have one polarity."

"The second polarity is Yin and Yang channels. When a channel that is on the Yin side of the body and has the word Yin in its name interacts with a Yang channel that is on the

Yang side of the body and has the word Yang in its name, this is another polarity. This is the Yin and Yang polarity.

"The last polarity is left and right. The channels exist on both sides of the body. So the channel that is on the right side is opposite a channel on the left side of the body."

"I think I get it. If we think about the channels, each channel can be said to be either a hand or foot channel and a Yin or Yang channel. We can see this in the names of the channels. When they interact with a different channel, we want one channel to be on the arm and the other on the foot, and we want one to be Yin and the other to be Yang. And for the last polarity, if the channel we want to interact with is on the right, then we would use the interacting channel on the left. Is that it?"

"That is very good, Sun. Everything you said is spot on. There is just one other thing to add. We only need two of the three polarities for channels to interact. This is why we have the last polarity of left and right, as this allows us to have interactions between more channels and have more ways of treating the body. We can classify the first two polarities as the main polarities:

Hand-Foot

Yin-Yang.

"And Left-Right as a secondary polarity. If a channel interaction already has the two main polarities in it, then we do not need to add the Left-Right polarity and can treat the patient on either side with the interacting channel. We have a few configurations of this:

When a Hand Yin channel interacts with a Foot Yang channel, the two basic polarities are met and can be treated on either side.

When an Arm Yang channel interacts with a Foot Yin channel, the two basic polarities are met and can be treated on either side.

When a Hand Yang channel interacts with a Hand Yin channel, there is only one basic polarity, so we need to treat on the opposite side.

When a Foot Yang channel interacts with a Foot Yin channel, there is only one basic polarity, so we need to treat on the opposite side.

When a Hand Yang channel interacts with a Foot Yang channel, there is only one basic polarity, so we need to treat on the opposite side.

When a Hand Yin channel interacts with a Foot Yin channel, there is only one basic polarity, so we need to treat on the opposite side."

"OK," said Sun. "This seems a bit confusing, but I am sure it will become clear as we see the channel interaction systems. Let me see if I can put all this together.

"For channels to interact they need to have a similarity. This similarity can be either a similarity of space, time, or sunlight. There are three systems that use the space similarity, two that use the time similarity, and one that uses the sunlight similarity. Once we have the similarity, there also needs to be at least two polarities. The polarities are Hand-Foot, Yin-Yang, and Left-Right.

"Some systems won't need to use Left-Right because they will already have the first two polarities present."

"That's it, Sun. A very good summary indeed."

PART III

SYSTEMS OF CHANNEL INTERACTIONS

Space-Based Channel Interactions

CHAPTER 10

WHERE EXACTLY
ARE WE?

Dinners with Sun's grandparents were normally light and easy to eat. There was always rice and that would be accompanied by lots of vegetables and a little fish or meat. This evening's meal was quite different. When Sun walked into the dining room, they saw a whole spread of some of their favorite things on the table. There were the dumplings that Grandmother Terra made with shrimps, there was a big plate of steaming noodles with fried egg and vegetables, and, best of all, there were many desserts. There was chocolate cake and carrot cake, and all the fruit you could imagine. Sun was surprised to see all these different foods on the table. They asked, "What is going on? Are we celebrating something today?"

Grandfather Terra responded, "Well, we decided to have a celebration of nothing in particular. Both your grandmother and myself feel a lot of joy at the moment with you staying with us and so we decided to allow our joy to be expressed by making some of your favorite things. So, in fact, we are celebrating you, Sun. And there is nothing more joyful than enjoying a nice meal with family and friends. Remember when we said that the emotions all have functions and that joy's function is connection? Well, we are honoring joy by creating a setting that helps us to connect more."

Sun had a big grin and was very touched. Their grandparents really knew how to make them feel special and loved. "Thank you very much, Grandmother Terra and Grandfather Terra. This is very nice, and I feel very happy that I get to spend my summer with you too. Now we should probably start eating as there is a lot of connecting to do."

The three of them ate until they were pleasantly full. None of them ate more than their body had asked for so they didn't feel heavy. They all knew that what didn't get eaten today would be lunch tomorrow, so none of the wonderful food would go to waste. After they had finished eating and cleaning up, Sun asked if they could talk a bit more about the channel interactions. And as they were all in a good mood, of course they did.

Sun started, "I know that we will start looking at the different systems of how the channels interact, but I wanted to make sure I understood something first. Today you mentioned that there are three systems based on space. I would just like to review this before we start talking about the actual interactions."

"Of course, Sun," said Grandmother Terra. "What would you like to review?"

"The idea of placements. Which channels are in which placements and why? I think I understood most of it, but I would like to have a quick review just to make sure."

"Of course. Let's start by remembering how the channels are organized. That should speak to most of your doubts. There are 12 channels, and each channel exists on both sides of the body. Right and left. When we look at the body in relationship to channels, we can talk about:

Upper limbs: hands and arms

Lower limbs: feet and legs

The torso

The head.

"The limbs are the most important in understanding how the channels are related to different positions.

"If we take the upper limb, we first divide it into a Yin side and a Yang side. The Yin side is the part that gets less sunlight, and the Yang side gets more sunlight.

"Once we have these two hemispheres, we then divide each hemisphere into three sections:

Front

Middle

Back.

"So, we now have six different segments on the arm:

Yin front

Yang front

Yin middle

Yang middle

Yin back

Yang back.

"Do you remember this?"

"Yes. That was how we first saw the channels before we added the Chinese names and the organs. We talked about the fact that each channel occupies a vertical segment of the body. It was either on the Yin side or the Yang side, and either in the front, middle, or back."

"That's exactly it, Sun. Well, when we are looking at the

first three systems of channel interactions, we use the position of the channels for the similarity. So, this means that the channels must occupy the same portion of the arm or leg—front, middle, back.

"Do you remember the names of the channels associated with each position?"

Sun nodded. "Yes I do. Let's start with the Yang side. On the Yang side of the arm or the leg, the section that gets the most sunlight is the back. The word Tai means most, so Tai Yang gets the most amount of sunlight on the Yang side of the body and is in the back.

"The area that gets the least amount of sunlight on the Yang side is the middle, and Shao means least or lesser amount of sun, so the middle channel is called Shao Yang.

"The last section is the front on the Yang side, and this gets the medium amount of sunlight and is called Ming, so Yang Ming is the name of the channel in the front of the Yang part of the body."

"That is exactly correct, Sun. And what about the Yin part of the body?"

"The Yin part of the body is slightly easier as it follows a more normal order. The front gets the most amount of sun so is called Tai Yin. The middle gets the medium amount of sun so is called Jue Yin. And the back gets the least amount of sun so is called Shao Yin."

Grandfather Terra nodded. "Perfect. Now let's put it altogether to understand the positions. In the front we have two channels. What are they?"

"In the front, there is the Yang Ming for the Yang side and the Tai Yin for the Yin side."

"And in the middle?"

"In the middle, there is the Shao Yang for the Yang side and the Jue Yin for the Yin side."

"And in the back?"

"In the back, there is the Tai Yang for the Yang side and the Shao Yin for the Yin side.

Front: Yang Ming and Tai Yin

Middle: Shao Yang and Jue Yin

Back: Tai Yang and Shao Yin."

Grandmother Terra responded, "That is perfect, Sun. So, when we talk about the first three systems, we use this. In these systems, the front channels interact with the other front channels, the middle channels interact with the other middle channels, and the back channels interact with the other back channels. The names of the systems are called:

System 1: Interior/Exterior or Biao/Li

System 2: Full Channels

System 3: Closed Circuit Channels.

"Each of these channel interaction systems has their own particularities and applications. And that we will start with tomorrow. We will start with System 1: Interior/Exterior."

Sun was happy. They felt ready for the next step. "That sounds good to me!"

And they all had a relaxing tea before bedtime.

CHAPTER 11

FOR EVERY YIN
THERE IS A YANG

System 1: Interior/Exterior or Biao/Li

Sun was looking out of their window after having done Qi Gong with their grandparents. Most of the time, after Qi Gong, Sun felt as if it was difficult to place themselves in time or space. They were not sure where they ended and where the outside world began. It was a pleasant feeling and opened many questions that were not yet formed in Sun's mind. They were just buds of questions waiting to flower. Sun just held them without being concerned, knowing they would open when they were ready. After a good daydream they went out to go for a walk with both grandparents. They had packed the leftover food from the previous day and were going to have a picnic in the forest.

Walking with the grandparents was always an interesting process. The grandparents would set a steady pace, after years of experience, that would allow them to walk for the whole day without getting too tired. It seemed as if it had taken years of practice to get that exact rhythm right. Sun was always surprised at how fit they were for their age. Sometimes Sun would be out of breath and the two of them would be walking as if there was no effort at all. Sun decided to learn as much from them as possible.

After a certain amount of time, the three sat down to enjoy their lunch. All the leftovers from the day before were put out on the blanket and they tucked in. Once they had finished eating, it was time for tea.

Sun jumped at the occasion and asked if they could start learning about the actual systems.

"Of course," replied Grandfather Terra. "Let's start with the first system: Interior/Exterior. This is perhaps the simplest system and most people who have studied acupuncture will have learned this in their studies.

"When we say Interior/Exterior we are referring to the Yin-Yang pair that is in each element. The Yang channel is more exterior, and the Yin channel is more interior. And these two channels can interact."

Grandmother Terra added, "We could also use the positions of the channels to understand this system. We will notice that the same position on the same limb is the Yin-Yang pairing from the elements."

Sun was a bit confused but then talked it out loud to make sure they understood. "So in each element, there is a Yin and a Yang pairing. They are:

Earth: Spleen and Stomach

Metal: Lung and Large Intestine

Water: Kidney and Bladder

Fire: Heart and Small Intestine

Wood: Liver and Gall Bladder

Heaven: Pericardium and Triple Warmer.

"Also, these pairings are in the same positions on the limbs:

Earth: Spleen and Stomach—front leg

Metal: Lung and Large Intestine—front arm

Water: Kidney and Bladder—back leg

Fire: Heart and Small Intestine—back arm

Wood: Liver and Gall Bladder—middle leg

Heaven: Pericardium and Triple Warmer—middle arm.

"So, you are saying that these channels have an interaction with each other?"

Grandfather Terra smiled. "Exactly that, Sun. If we want to treat a problem that is on one of the channels, we can use its Yin-Yang pairing to treat it. If we were to put this on the Unified Acupuncture Theory model we showed you, it would look like this image."

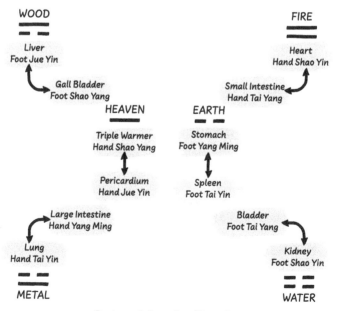

System 1: Interior/Exterior

Sun looked at the drawing and nodded. "So if, for example, I wanted to treat the Hand Shao Yang Triple Warmer channel, I would look for the Yin channel that is in the same element (heaven), which is the Hand Jue Yin Pericardium channel, and use that?"

"Perfect, Sun. Now we need to think about the rules of how channels interact to see how to apply this. Remember there needs to be one similarity based on space, time, or sunlight. What similarity is there here?"

"Well, we said that the elements occupy the same place on the limbs, so it must be that space is the similarity."

"Yes, and we also need at least two polarities. The two basic polarities are Yin/Yang and Hand/Foot and the third polarity that can be added is Left/Right. How many basic polarities does this channel relationship have?"

"There is a Yin channel interacting with a Yang channel, so that is one. But as the elements are on the same limbs then they do not have the Hand/Foot polarity. So only one."

"Exactly. Because there is only one basic polarity in this interaction, Yin/Yang, we must use the third polarity, Left/Right. This means that we need to treat on the opposite side of the problem. For example, if someone had pain on the right wrist on the Hand Yang Ming Large Intestine, what channel would you use to treat it and how?"

"Well, the Hand Yang Ming Large Intestine is in the front Yang position of the arm and is in the metal element. The channel that is in the front Yin position of the arm and also in the metal element is the Hand Tai Yin Lung. And as these are both in the arm, I need to use the third polarity, Left/Right. So, if the problem is on the right side, I would use the Left Tai Yin Lung channel. But I still do not know where on the channel I would place the needles."

Grandmother Terra answered, "That is absolutely correct, Sun. If the problem is on the right wrist on the Hand Yang

Ming Large Intestine channel, we would use the Hand Tai Yin Lung on the left side to treat it. Now we will include the holography we studied before. We will look for an image of the wrist on the Hand Tai Yin Lung channel. Look at the image and tell me where you would put the needles."

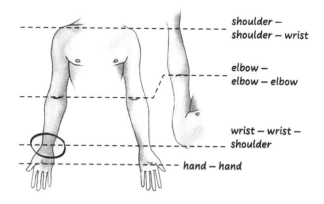

Sun looked and answered, "Well, I see that the wrist will image the wrist, as does the shoulder. So, I would put the needles in either the shoulder or the wrist on the left arm on the Hand Tai Yin Lung channel. How would I know which one to use, wrist or shoulder?"

"Well, first you are correct. The wrist and the shoulder both image the wrist. So, well done. Now we can think about which is the best choice for the needles. And to do this the first guide is called anatomical similarity. This means we are looking for similar structures in the place where we put the needles and the place we are interacting with.

"The Hand Yang Ming Large Intestine channel on the right wrist is a bony structure with lots of ligaments. So we then look at the Hand Tai Yin Lung channel on the left shoulder and the left wrist and see which area is more similar. A good way to do this is to first put your finger on the right wrist at the Hand Yang Ming Large Intestine area and feel around. Then put your finger on the left Hand Tai Yin Lung shoulder and wrist areas and ascertain which feels most alike."

Sun started touching their wrists and shoulder. After a good examination they said, "The wrist on the Hand Tai Yin Lung is more similar to the area of the Hand Yang Ming Large Intestine wrist than the shoulder is. So, I would use the wrist area of the Hand Tai Yin Lung to treat the opposite wrist area of the Hand Yang Ming Large Intestine."

"Perfect. So now we can treat a problem at the wrist. This is your first practical acupuncture treatment."

It was as if a light went on in Sun's mind. "Hold on. Is this why when I was smaller and would be playing and fell, you would massage another point on my body and the pain would go away?"

Grandfather Terra laughed. "You remember that, hmmm. Yes, that is what we were doing. You can use this with massage or just applying pressure on the point to get a similar response. However, using needles has a longer and deeper effect. In fact, you can also use this palpation technique if you aren't sure which image or system to use. You can palpate the possible treatments and see which one gets the best result first and then needle that point."

"You said that there are six systems. Does this system, Interior/Exterior, have any special uses or differences from the other systems?"

"That's a very good question. Every system will work with various degrees of success. And sometimes one system will work for a while and then it will work less well. That is normal. Each system does have its particular attributes which makes it perhaps more effective in certain situations. To understand this, we need to look at the system and how the channels interact in it.

"Let's start by looking at the system we just learned,

Interior-Exterior. If we examine it, we will find the following characteristics. Both the affected and the interacting channel are on the same limb and in the same position and both of them are part of the same element. So, these are the characteristics that can help us to understand the types of interactions this system might work better for.

"Both channels are on the same limbs, which also means they pass through the same articulations:

Wrist—elbow—shoulder.

"Or:

Ankle—knee—hip.

"And as we saw with our example, the wrist of the Hand Tai Yin Lung was very similar to the Hand Yang Ming Hand. This is especially true in the wrists and the ankles. So, one specialty of System 1 is that it is very good for treating wrists and ankles. It is also good for elbows and knees too. When it comes to shoulders and hips, it can be useful but may not have the most anatomical similarities."

Sun took it all in. That made good sense. The wrists and the knees were much more similar on the Yin and Yang sides of the body than the other joints. Then Sun asked, "What about the element concept that you raised earlier? How does that play a role in why System 1 Interior/Exterior may be used?"

"That's another good question. So far, we have only talked about the channels and the basic ideas of the organs. In Chinese medicine, there are many other aspects that can be included. This includes the functions associated with each of the organs and, by extension, the elements. Remember we talked last year about how the elements can be used as a classification system? Each element has a type of quality, and when we look at a group of things, we can put each thing in the group in one of the elements. We did this when we talked about the emotions. We said that the emotion of sadness is associated with the metal element. We can use this in our choice of systems also.

"Let's say we have a patient who has a problem on the upper thigh on the Foot Tai Yin Spleen channel. Based on System 1, how would you treat it?"

"First I would look at which channel interacts with Foot Tai Yin Spleen. That would be the Foot Yang Ming Stomach. Then I would look for the image of the upper thigh on the Foot Yang Ming Stomach channel. This would be also the upper thigh but on the opposite leg."

"Excellent. And that is a very good treatment because both upper thigh regions are full of muscle and have similar anatomical structures. Now we can also say that the patient has abdominal cramps and digestion issues. The earth element is also associated with digestion issues. And let's also say the patient overthinks things and is always analyzing things. This is associated with the earth element. So not only are the anatomical similarities useful but also the functions and other characteristics of the element can be used. And System 1 is the only system where both the affected and the interacting channel are in the same element. So, this is the other specialty of System 1 Interior/Exterior."

Sun was silent for a moment, then said, "Let me see if I got the whole idea of System 1. The system is called Interior/Exterior. It matches the Yin and Yang channels of the same element together. These channels also share the same limb and position.

Front Hand Tai Yin Lung with Front Hand Yang Ming Large Intestine—metal

Front Foot Tai Yin Spleen with Front Foot Yang Ming Stomach—earth

Middle Hand Jue Yin Pericardium with Middle Hand
   Shao Yang Triple Warmer—heaven

Middle Foot Jue Yin Liver with Middle Foot Shao Yang
   Gall Bladder—wood

Back Hand Shao Yin Heart with Back Hand Tai Yang
   Small Intestine—fire

Back Foot Shao Yin Kidney with Back Foot Tai Yang
   Bladder—water.

"As these interactions are on the same limb (Hand or Foot) the channels only have one basic polarity (Yin/Yang) so they are used on the opposite sides of each other.

"This system has two specialties. The first is that it is good for wrists and ankles and also elbows and knees. The second is that when the functions—emotions, organ functions, or other associations—that are assigned to the element are affected, this system can be useful. Is that it?"

Both the grandparents smiled and said in unison, "Yes, Sun. That is it."

CHAPTER 12

ONE LONG PATHWAY

System 2: Full Channels or Shared Channel Names

Sun looked at both grandparents with a big smile. "I know that we normally talk in small chunks, but I was wondering if we could continue directly with the next system. I feel as if I am in a good learning mode and want to continue."

Grandfather Terra's expression was one of accepting an inevitability when he responded, "Yes, Sun. We can see that you are in a good learning space, and we can continue. But also be aware that even if the mood for learning is there, it will still take time to integrate what you have learned. So, it is good to not bite off too much to chew, otherwise you will be chewing for longer. We agree that we can continue with the next system. As it is also based on space, it won't be too much more to digest."

"Great," Sun said, with a big grin.

Grandmother Terra began, "We saw with the previous system that we used the elements to find the relationship. If the channels were associated with the same channel, then they could interact, and this led to what we called the Interior/Exterior relationship. For this relationship, we will use what we call the Full Channels. Remember that each channel has a name that has four parts:

Part 1: Hand or Foot—where the channel either begins or ends

Part 2: The Chinese Word, Tai, Shao, Jue, Ming—how much sunlight it gets

Part 3: Yin or Yang—which aspect of the body the channel is on

Part 4: The Organ—the internal organ that is associated with the channel.

"For this system, we will be using parts 2 and 3 for the similarity. When the channel has the same Chinese word and is on the same aspect of the body, they will interact. Which means that:

Tai Yang will interact with Tai Yang

Yang Ming will interact with Yang Ming

Shao Yang will interact with Shao Yang

Tai Yin will interact with Tai Yin

Jue Yin will interact with Jue Yin

Shao Yin will interact with Shao Yin.

"One will either start or finish in the hand and the other in the foot."

Sun thought about this for a moment. "OK, I see. So, it is the channel names and Yin-Yang polarity that are the similarities. How does this relate to space? As Grandfather Terra said this earlier, I would like to understand what he meant by that."

Grandfather Terra answered, "Well, the names of the

channels explain how much sunlight each channel gets. Remember that the channels are the vertical segments of the body. And these vertical segments that get the same amount of sun also occupy the same position on the Yin or Yang side of the body. For example, the Tai Yang means the most amount of sunlight on the Yang side of the body. The positions on the back of the arms and the back of the legs both get the most amount of sunlight on the Yang side of the body. So Tai Yang occupies this back position in both the legs and the arms. The Hand Tai Yang Small Intestine, which is in the back of the Yang side of the arm, and the Foot Tai Yang Bladder, which is on the back of the leg, will interact with each other. They both have the same name—Tai—which means most amount of sunlight, and they are both on the Yang side of the body and they are both in the back."

"Yes, I see what you meant now. In fact, we could use the position and the polarity to explain the interaction. Back Yang in the arm interacts with back Yang in the leg. The Chinese name is making the same reference, but adding the idea of sunlight."

"Exactly."

"So, to make things simple, we could say:

Back Yang hand interacts with back Yang foot

Middle Yang hand interacts with middle Yang foot

Front Yang hand interacts with front Yang foot.

"And it is the same for the Yin:

Back Yin hand interacts with back Yin foot

Middle Yin hand interacts with middle Yin foot

Front Yin hand interacts with front Yin foot."

"Yes. And as the positions have the same channel name, we

call this system Full Channels, meaning that two channels that have the same name can interact. If we were to use the channel names here it would be, for the Yang channels:

Hand Tai Yang interacts with Foot Tai Yang

Hand Yang Ming interacts with Foot Yang Ming

Hand Shao Yang interacts with Foot Shao Yang.

"And for the Yin channels:

Hand Tai Yin interacts with Foot Tai Yin

Hand Jue Yin interacts with Foot Jue Yin

Hand Shao Yin interacts with Foot Shao Yin.

"And on the Unified Acupuncture Theory model it looks like this image."

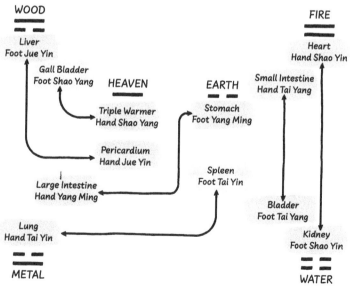

System 2: Full Channels

Sun looked at the image for a while and then commented, "I see. And this is different from the previous system of channel interactions because we are not staying in the same element. Also, I notice something else. The Yin and Yang channel of an element are both interacting with another element. I mean that when I look at the metal element, Hand Tai Yin Lung and Hand Yang Ming Large Intestine are both interacting with the earth element. Hand Tai Yin Lung and Hand Yang Ming Large Intestine are both metal, and Foot Tai Yin Spleen and Foot Yang Ming Stomach are both earth. So here, metal is interacting with earth."

Grandmother Terra nodded. "That is a very good observation. Each position has two elements associated with it.

Front: metal and earth

Middle: heaven and wood

Back: fire and water.

"One element is associated with channels in the leg and the other in the arm. And this system—System 2 Full Channels—has the Yang of one element interacting with the Yang of the other element.

"So, we understand the similarity that is based on space. How about the polarities? How many of the two base polarities are there? Remember they are Hand-Foot and Yin-Yang."

Sun answered, "Well, we have already said that one is a hand channel and the other is a foot channel, so that is one polarity. However, both the channels in this system have the same name so they are both the same Yin-Yang polarity. Hand Tai Yang is interacting with Foot Tai Yang. They are both Yang. I see. There is only one base polarity in this system."

"Exactly. And as there is only one base polarity, we need to add the third polarity system Left-Right. So, this system means that we treat on the opposite side of the problem. If the person has a problem on the right side, we will use the left interacting channel to treat it. OK, I think we understand the basics of the system now, so how about an example?

"A person has pain in the left leg. The pain is at the part we call the Achilles tendon, and it is on the Yin part of the tendon. Let's go through the process together.

"First, we need to identify the channel where the problem is. What channel is affected, Sun?" Grandmother Terra asked, while pointing to the inside area of the Achilles tendon on the left leg just above the ankle.

Sun looked at what she was pointing at and said, "It's at the back, on the leg, and on the Yin side. So, it is the Back Yin Foot channel. This area gets the least amount of sunlight on the Yin part of the body, so it is called Shao. So, the Foot Shao Yin Kidney channel."

"That is correct. So now if we want to use System 2 Full Channels, which channel interacts with Foot Shao Yin Kidney?"

"Foot Shao Yin Kidney is in the back of the leg on the Yin side. System 2 uses the same position but on the opposite limb (above/below). It is also the channel that has the same Chinese name—the Hand (opposite foot) Shao Yin and it is associated with the Heart. The Hand Shao Yin Heart channel is the interacting channel for System 2."

"Very good, Sun. Now it is time to image the problem from the sick or affected channel to the interacting channel. The problem on the Foot Shao Yin Kidney channel is just above the ankle on the tendon. Where could we look for this on the Hand Shao Yin Heart channel?"

"This is the more difficult part for me to imagine. Let me

try to think my way through it. The lower limb mirrors the upper limb. The joints are the reference for the mirroring. Wrist to ankle, elbow to knee, and shoulder to hip. If the problem is above the ankle, I would use the ankle as my reference and look at the wrist."

Grandfather Terra nodded. "Yes, Sun, that is almost it. We need to now adjust the image for the exact place of the problem. In this case, it is just above the ankle, so we say it is proximal to the ankle. We move the same distance away from the wrist in the same direction (proximal) along the channel. The image is slightly proximal from the wrist on the Hand Shao Yin Heart channel."

"Yes, that makes sense. And what about the other image? When the shoulder images the wrist? Could we also use near the shoulder to image the Achilles tendon?"

"Good question, Sun. Yes, we could use the shoulder, and we would have to adapt the image to target the affected area. This means we would be slightly distal (further away from the body on the shoulder). Now which do you think is a better treatment, remembering the idea of anatomical similarity?"

"The shoulder area on the Hand Shao Yin Heart channel is at the armpit. So first of all, I think it would be smelly, but more than that it does not feel like the tendons. With the wrist area, I can feel a tendon under my finger when I touch there, so I would say the wrist is a better image."

Both grandparents laughed. Grandmother Terra said, "Besides the smelly reason of the armpit, you are right. The area near the wrist is a closer image of the anatomy of the tendon on the leg than the armpit. Here, look at this picture to see the imaging."

left arm   left arm   right arm   left leg   left leg   left leg

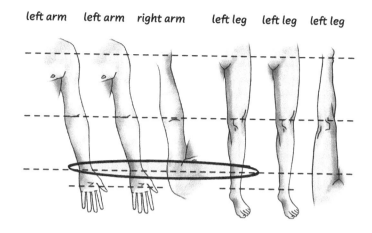

Sun saw the image and then had a thought. "What if the problem on the tendon is on both sides of the tendon—the Yin and the Yang side?"

"That's a very good question. In the first instance, we saw that it was on the Yin side, the Foot Shao Yang Kidney channel, and we used the Full Channel relationship with the Hand Shao Yin Heart channel. Now let's add the Yang side of the tendon. What channel passes through that area?"

"So the back Yang channel of the leg. That would be the Foot Tai Yang Bladder."

"Very good. And now, using the same system, System 2 Full Channels, what channel interacts with the Foot Tai Yang Bladder?"

"This system is keeping the position and the polarity but changing the limb. Instead of the leg, I would look for the same channel on the arm. The Hand Tai Yang Small Intestine is my answer."

"Good. And now what image would you use?"

"I think it would also be the wrist."

"That is the answer to your question, Sun. If both sides of the tendon are affected then we need to interact with both channels that pass over that area. We could use System 2 for this. For the Foot Shao Yin Kidney side of the problem on the tendon we would choose the Hand Shao Yin Heart, and for the Foot Tai Yang Bladder side of the tendon we can use the Hand Tai Yang Small Intestine channel. And remember that System 2 only has one base polarity, Hand-Foot, and we need to add the Left-Right polarity. So, we would treat on the opposite hand of the injured tendon. And if the problem is on both sides, we would treat on both arms.

"Now that is only if we use System 2. We still have four more systems to explore. We might find a different treatment—one channel that interacts with both the Foot Shao Yin Kidney and the Foot Tai Yang Bladder—and use only that channel, but for now we would treat with this."

"That makes sense," said Sun. "So, if I want to sum up this system, the system is called Full Channels. This is because the foot and hand channels that are interacting both have the same name and are the same channel, but one is in the foot and the other in the hand. As they have the same name, they also occupy the same position: front, middle, and back. They are also on the same Yin or Yang polarity. This means that they need to be used on the opposite side as they have only one base polarity, Hand-Foot."

"We could not have summed it up better, Sun."

CHAPTER 13

Crossing Paths

System 3: Closed Circuit Channels

The hike and the talk had left all three with a feeling of accomplishment. When they got home, they all went to the porch for a hard-earned rest with afternoon tea and the delicious desserts they had left over from the day before.

Before the last sip of tea, Sun smiled and said, "We saw two systems that were based on space today. And there are three systems that are based on space. What is this last space-based system?"

Grandfather Terra shook his head. "Ever the student wanting to know more. Well, as you have digested everything so far, we can continue. The last space-based system is called Closed Circuit Channels. Now the name is not very descriptive until we see all the space-based systems together, but it is the name of the system so we will use it. Let's first recap the first two systems we saw and see if we can figure out the third one.

System 1 was Interior/Exterior. The Yin and Yang of the same position on the same limb interacted with each other.

System 2 was Full Channels. The Yin and Yin or the Yang

and Yang of the arm and limb in the same position interacted with each other.

"What do you think the third system is?"

Sun thought for a moment. "Well, the third system is a space-based system. So, the position of front, middle, or back needs to be respected. If we take just one position to think about it—the front, for example—let's see.

"For the front channels, we have already seen that:

- the front hand Yin interacts with the front hand Yang (System 1: Interior/Exterior)

- the front hand Yin interacts with the front foot Yin (System 2: Full Channels).

"That leaves only one channel in the front that the front arm Yin channel hasn't interacted with yet. The front foot Yang. So, I would think this system would have that interaction."

Grandmother Terra nodded. "That's exactly it, Sun. In this system we will see that we stay in the same position but change the limb and the Yin-Yang polarity. So, as you said, the front arm Yin channel will interact with the front foot Yang channel.

"We keep the same position—front, middle, back—and add the two polarities. So, the correspondences are as follows:

Front:

Hand Tai Yin Lung—Foot Yang Ming Stomach

Hand Yang Ming Large Intestine—Foot Tai Yin Spleen

Middle:

Hand Jue Yin Pericardium—Foot Shao Yang Gall Bladder

Hand Shao Yang Triple Warmer—Foot Jue Yin Liver

Back:

Hand Shao Yin Heart—Foot Tai Yang Bladder

Hand Tai Yang Small Intestine—Foot Shao Yin Kidney.

"You can look at the model to see them."

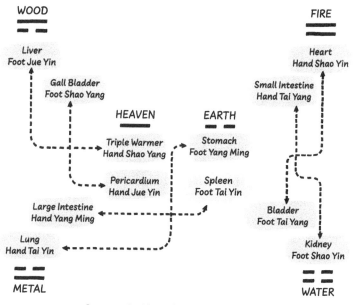

System 3: Closed Circuit Channels

Sun studied the image. "So, this is the last connection with the position of the channels. We change the limb and the Yin-Yang but keep the position. Why are the lines dotted here and not solid?"

"Very observant. The dotted lines are telling us about the polarity of the system. Remember that we need one similarity and at least two polarities. What are the similarity and the polarities of this system?"

"Well, the similarity is space. The interacting channels are both either in the front, middle, or back. For the polarities, let's see. We have an arm channel interacting with a foot channel. So that is one polarity. There is a Yin channel interacting with a Yang channel, so that is another polarity. So, these are the two basic polarities in this system."

"Exactly. Both the basic polarities of above and below and Yin and Yang are present. This means that we do not have to add the Left-Right polarity. So, we can treat the affected channel with the interacting channel on the same side as the problem or the opposite side. And the dotted lines help us to see this. When there is a dotted line, it means that the system has the two basic polarities and can be used either side. When the line is solid, it means that the two basic polarities are not present and only one of the basic polarities is there, so we have to use the opposite side.

"Solid line means opposite side must be used. Dotted line means either side can be used."

"Oh, I see. The dotted or solid lines are there to help us quickly remember the polarity situation of the system. That makes sense. Can we try using this system?"

Grandfather Terra pointed at his left foot. He said that he had pain between the big toe and the second toe, on the top of the foot. "Here is my pain. What is the affected channel and how would you treat it?"

Sun thought and then answered. "The affected channel is the Foot Jue Yin Liver channel. This is the middle channel on the Yin side of the leg. To use System 3 Closed Circuit Channels, we would stay in the same position—middle—and change the limb and the Yin-Yang polarity.

"Foot to hand and Yin to Yang using the middle channels would take me to the hand Yang middle channel, which is the Hand Shao Yang Triple Warmer.

"Now how to image it? The foot images to the hand. And the top of the foot images to the palm and the back of the hand. So, I would look for a similar place on the hand between the bones of the fingers."

"Perfect, Sun. These bones have names. On the foot, they are the metatarsal bones, and on the hand, they are the metacarpal bones. So, we would treat the problem between the first and second metatarsal bones on the Foot Jue Yin Liver channel with the area between the fourth and fifth metacarpal bones on the Hand Shao Yang Triple Warmer channel. Now which side would we use, remembering that the problem was on my left foot?"

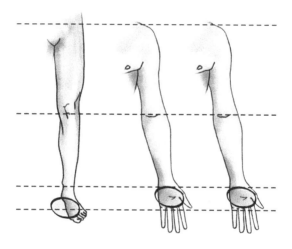

"We could use either side as this is System 3 Closed Circuit Channels, and has both of the base polarities: above/below and Yin/Yang. So could you now explain the name?"

"Yes, but first some more tea."

CHAPTER 14

GATHERING ALL THE MATTER

Space-Based Systems Compared

Grandmother Terra sipped the tea and looked at Sun. She was enjoying how much her grandchild loved learning. She saw herself as a small child when she looked at Sun. Sun's curiosity and ability to understand systems felt like a mirror of herself. She knew that Grandfather Terra felt the same about this child. And they also worried about Sun. Sun did not have the same vision of the world as most of their classmates and other children their age. Sun could grasp ideas that were difficult for even adults to get, and Sun got them with ease and clarity. And this led to the worry. Sun was beyond their years when it came to understanding, yet they were still a child. They still had a lot of emotional growth ahead of them. Using their intellect to navigate their emotions could lead Sun to over-rely on their mind and detach from their feelings. Grandmother Terra knew this all too well, as this was her road. It was not until she was much older that she had been ready to start understanding her own emotions. The two grandparents had talked about this often and even raised their concerns to Sun's parents. There was little they could do to help Sun navigate these difficult times except to continue to be there for Sun and model their own interactions with their emotions.

Grandmother Terra asked Sun, "Before we continue, and we will continue with understanding the name of the third system, can I ask you something, Sun?"

Sun said, "Sure. Ask away."

"If you were to imagine that all the information we are talking about and the knowledge you are getting was stored somewhere in your body, where would you say it was stored?"

"That is a strange question. Hmm, let me think. Well, I guess I would say it is all in my head. Yes, my head is where I keep it all."

"Yes, we keep our knowledge in our head. And if we were to also look for a place in the body, where would it be in the body? For example, think about the channel systems we have learned so far. When you hold the image of them in your head, can you feel a part of your body that isn't the head tingling or being active in some way? Take a moment, take a few breaths, and try to feel where it might be."

Sun breathed deeply, trying to feel something. "I am not sure I understand. The knowledge is in my head. That is where it is."

"OK. Let's try this. When you are learning about the systems, or anything, from me and your grandfather, there is a feeling in your body as well as the knowledge entering your mind. As we talk about the systems now, I would like you to try to feel your body while we listen. It may be similar to when we do the Qi Gong. There are feelings in the body. We don't have to put words to them, but we can notice they are there. Try to be aware of where in your body you are responding to what we are talking about.

"So, the first three systems. They are all based on space. We have:

System 1: Interior/Exterior

System 2: Full Channels

System 3: Closed Circuit Channels.

"As they are all based on space, they all use the same position as their similarity:

Front channels interact with the other front channels

Middle channels interact with the other middle channels

Back channels interact with the other back channels.

"And if we look at the UAT model, we will see that each of the positions has two elements attached to it:

Front: metal and earth

Middle: heaven and wood

Back: fire and water.

"And in each position, there is one element that has channels in the arm and one in the leg. Do you remember why the element will have channels in either the arm or the leg?"

"Yes. The foot channels can only be in elements where the bottom line of the image describing the Yin-Yang of the element is a broken Yin line. And for arm channels, the bottom line is a solid Yang channel."

"Great. So, each position has one element that is associated with channels in the hand and one element that has channels associated in the foot.

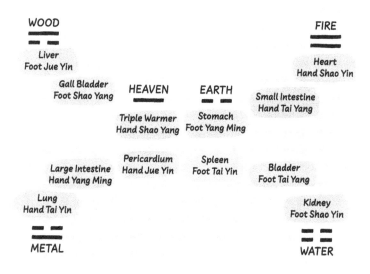

"And each of the space-based systems will describe an interaction between the four channels that are in each position.

> System 1: Interior/Exterior we stay in the element and the same limb. We move from Yin to Yang or Yang to Yin.

> System 2: Full Channels we stay on the same polarity of Yin or Yang, but we change the limb and the element.

"So, if we look at only Systems 1 and 2, we will see this:

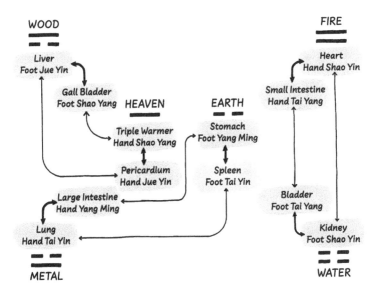

"We have connected the two elements that make up each position using System 2 Full Channels, where the Yin hand and Yin foot interact and the Yang hand and the Yang foot interact. When we add System 3 Closed Circuit Channels, we see this:

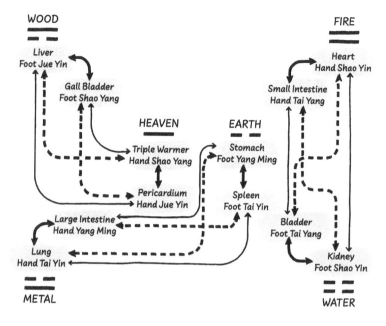

"We see that the third system, Closed Circuit Channels, connects the arm element's hand Yin channel with the leg element's foot Yang channel. And it connects the arm element's Yang channel with the leg element's Yin channel. This means that all the channels in a position can interact with all the other channels that are in the same position. And System 3 completes a closed circuit of these channels, where they can all interact with each other, thus the name Closed Circuit Channels."

Sun was silent for a moment and then responded, "I see. The name Closed Circuit Channels describes how System 3 completes the space-based systems and they create a continuous loop between them. It reminds me of a square where all the four corners can connect with all the other corners.

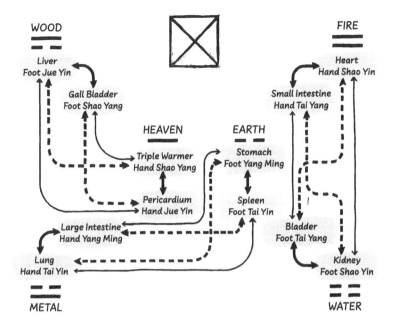

"I have another question. When should I choose one of these systems? And how to choose among them?"

Grandfather Terra responded, "That is an excellent question. And one that has a few answers. The first is a general answer to this question for all the systems. We use anatomical similarities. As we saw when we looked at Systems 1 and 2 and were comparing the images, the wrist was a better image of the wrist than the shoulder as it had a more similar anatomical structure. We would say the same for the systems.

"A second answer would be about polarity. Systems 1 and 2 both only have one basic polarity so they must be used on the opposite side, whereas System 3 has both basic polarities so can be used on either side. This can be important when we use certain styles of acupuncture that limit where we can needle or when there are counter-indications for needling certain segments of the body.

"And a third reason can be specific to the nature of the relationship to the problem. We saw that the first system is the only system where we stay within the same element. We have the Yin channel of the element interacting with the Yang channel of the element. This means that the other elements are not involved with the treatment. All the other systems use different elements, and we can analyze how they interact when we study the elements more in depth, but that is not what we are doing here."

Sun interrupted, "Hold on. I feel like you are going too fast and giving too much information at the same time."

Grandmother Terra smiled. "Where did you feel that, Sun? Where did your body tell you that it felt discomfort?"

Sun closed their eyes and breathed. "It was in my stomach. I felt my stomach get tighter."

Grandmother Terra nodded. "Good. So, you felt your body tell you that something was not OK. That is what I was saying before. We will get back to reminding Grandfather Terra about his tendency to lecture in a moment," she said, winking at her partner.

"Now Sun, try to feel more into what you felt in your stomach. Can you describe it a little more?"

"There is tightness and a heaviness. Also, there is a feeling of needing to do something. It was as if a spring was winding up and when I spoke it unsprang."

"That is an interesting description of the feeling. Now, do you remember the emotions we talked about on the previous hike? What emotion do you think you might be feeling?"

"Well, it feels tight and spring-like. Like a bamboo that was bent down and wanted to spring back straight. So that is like a tree. And trees are wood. Could it be anger? But this is not what I think anger would be."

"I would agree with you that it is anger. This is healthy anger. You felt as if you were being overwhelmed mentally and you needed to protect yourself. Anger is about protecting yourself and this is exactly what you did. You stopped Grandfather Terra from assaulting you with his exuberance. So, let us take a moment to thank your body for feeling this and taking a pause from the learning as it was getting too much.

"I want you to remember this as an experience that you can learn from. I see myself in you, as I was similar when I was young—not as intuitive and bright as you, but similar. From my experience, I want to help you learn to feel your body and to listen to it. People like us, who feel that we need to understand everything, have a tendency to not listen to our bodies. We identify with the mind, which feels like a safer place than the body. As you go out into the world and are confronted with many new experiences and emotions, if you practice listening to your body and how you feel, it will help you better understand yourself and your emotions. And that is the end of my lecture. Let's go back to the systems."

Sun was smiling. They had understood that their body felt the emotion before they were aware of it. And it made sense to them that being aware of their body will help them understand all the weird things they feel sometimes. "OK, let's get back to calming Grandfather Terra now."

Grandfather Terra was laughing. "Thank you both for your support. Well, Sun, let's say this. When we want to understand which is the best system to use, we use the same logic as the images. First, we look for the most similar anatomical structure. Then we can also take into account the nature of the channel interactions using our understanding of the elements and other aspects of Chinese medicine. And we can always use palpation if we are not sure."

"I think I get it. It is like saying that all the systems will work, but some systems have more similar anatomical similarities at certain areas than others. So, palpating the areas will help to find those similarities.

"Now I feel that there is an opening in my chest, as if a light is coming out. I think this might be joy as I am connecting to the information and both of you."

"And with that perfect summary of what you are feeling, we will end for today," Grandmother Terra said with a beaming smile.

TIME-BASED CHANNEL INTERACTIONS

CHAPTER 15

EVERY CHANNEL WILL HAVE ITS HOUR (OR TWO)

An Explanation of the Biorhythm Clock

Sun woke up refreshed. They had slept well as their body, mind, and spirit had a good workout the previous day. The body had walked on the long hike, their mind had absorbed the three systems based on space, and their spirit had worked with emotions. It was a complete day and Sun hoped today would be the same.

Sun enjoyed the ritual aspect of life at their grandparents' place. Every action and event had a flow to it and also something to mark the change. The rituals of eating, gardening, and even talking felt very comforting to Sun. And the day's rituals flowed along until finally Sun found themselves sitting on the porch with a cup of tea about to start the next lesson.

Grandmother Terra started. "How are you today, Sun? How do you feel after learning the first three systems of channel interactions?"

"I am excited. I feel it in my chest. It is as if a blue light is getting ready to shine somewhere."

"Great. Well expressed. And how did you feel about the three systems yesterday? Were you able to integrate them all?"

"I think so. They are all based on space, which means that the position of the channel is the common feature in all three systems. If I were to sum it up, all the front channels interact with each other, all the middle channels interact with each other, and all the back channels interact with each other.

The front channels are Tai Yin and Yang Ming

The middle channels are Jue Yin and Shao Yang

The back channels are Shao Yin and Tai Yang.

"And:

System 1: Interior/Exterior has the same limb but different Yin-Yang polarity

System 2: Full Channels has the same Yin-Yang polarity but different limb

System 3: Closed Circuit Channels changes both the Yin-Yang polarity and the limb."

"That is a perfect summary, Sun. So, now we are ready to start on the next group of systems. Do you remember what they are based on?"

"They are based on time, and I assume that means the channel clock that we looked at last year, where each channel is associated with a two-hour period. If so, could we do a quick reminder of how the clock is created? I found it really interesting."

"You are correct Sun, it is the channel clock, and we will do a review of it before we start looking at the time-based systems.

"The 24-hour cycle of the sun is what governs the clock. And of Yin and Yang, Yang is more associated with the presence of the sun, so the key to understanding the placement of the channels on the clock is the Yang channels. There are three full Yang channels:

Tai Yang

Yang Ming

Shao Yang.

"And these names refer to how much sunlight the channels get:

Tai Yang gets the most amount of sun

Yang Ming gets the medium amount of sun

Shao Yang gets the least amount of sun.

"We start by taking a 24-hour day and we divide it into three eight-hour segments, one for each Yang channel:

11am–7pm

7pm–3am

3am–11am

"If we put these two ideas together, we would associate them as:

11am–7pm: most amount of sun—Tai Yin

7pm–3am: least amount of sun—Shao Yin

3am–11am.: medium amount of sun—Yang Ming.

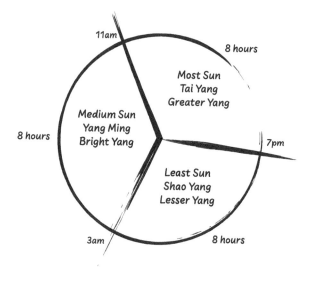

"In these eight-hour segments, we put the Yang channel in the four-hour middle of the segment:

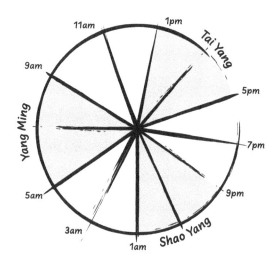

"If we think about the flow of Qi in the body, we know that the Qi from Yang flows down from the sun to the earth. So, the Qi first starts in the hands, goes to the face, and then goes down to the feet. This means that we put the hand aspect of the channel first, and the foot aspect second. So, we put the hand aspect in the first two hours of the middle four-hour segment, and the foot aspect in the second two-hour segment.

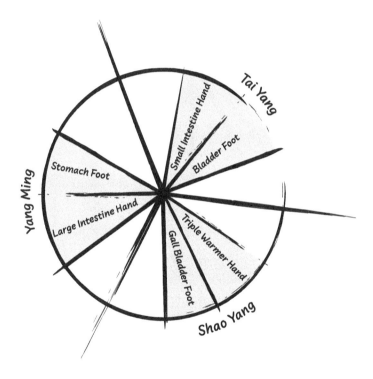

"Now to add the Yin channels we split them up and do not have the hand of one channel next to the foot of the same channel. Instead, we use the Interior/Exterior relationship from System 1, and put the Yin channel that has the interior/exterior relationship with the Yang channel next to it.

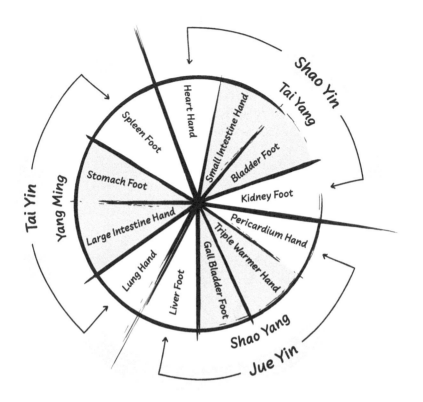

"That is the quick summary from last year."

Sun nodded. "Yes, I remember all that. I remember that we also went much further with the construction. It is one of my favorite theories from last summer because it is so complete. So, I understand the placement of the channels where they are, but what does it mean that each channel has a specific time? Isn't the Qi flowing all the time through all the channels?"

Grandfather Terra responded, "Yes, the Qi is flowing through the channels all the time and in all directions. There are also times where the Qi flows more fluidly than others, with more power. It is like the ocean, the tides, and the currents. There is always water everywhere. And there are certain currents that move the water. These currents are like the channels. Between the currents there is still water and between the channels there is still Qi. The ocean also has tides. These are the big movements of when it rises and falls. High tide is when the area of water is at its highest point, and low tide is when it is at its lowest point. The channels also have this tidal flow. When we refer to the two-hour period associated with a channel, that is like its high tide, and it has the most Qi in it compared to the other times of day."

"That makes sense. So, there is Qi always everywhere, like water in the ocean. The channels are like currents that move the Qi around, and the hours of the clock are like the high tide."

"Perfect. That is it. The channel clock is usually written with the channel abbreviations to make it easier. Here are the abbreviations so that if you see the clock in an acupuncture book you will understand it:

LU: Hand Tai Yin Lung

LI: Hand Yang Ming Large Intestine

ST: Foot Yang Ming Stomach

SP: Foot Tai Yin Spleen

HT: Hand Shao Yin Heart

SI: Hand Tai Yang Small Intestine

BL: Foot Tai Yang Bladder

KI or KID: Foot Shao Yin Kidney

PC: Hand Jue Yin Pericardium

TW or SJ or TE: Hand Shao Yang Triple Warmer (SJ = San Jiao; TE = Triple Energizer)

GB: Foot Shao Yang Gall Bladder

LV or LIV: Foot Jue Yin Liver.

"So the clock is often shown like this image."

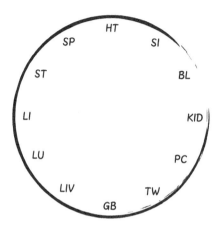

"OK. I can see this. So how do we use this to understand the channel interactions?"

Grandmother Terra smiled. "First, drink your tea."

CHAPTER 16

FRIENDLY NEIGHBORS

System 4: Biorhythm Neighbors

Sun drank the tea in one gulp and then made a point of making a loud "ah" to show that they had finished it. Both grandparents laughed. "OK. The first system based on time," said Grandfather Terra, "is called Biorhythm Neighbors. And the system states that any channels that are next to another channel on the biorhythm clock can interact with each other. Think of it as if all the channels are out for dinner at a big round table—like when the whole family went for Chinese last year and we all sat around the round table. It had a lazy Susan on the table that spun around so the food could be shared."

"I remember that. With Grandmother Terra we tried to spin it fast enough to see if the shrimp could fly across the room. My parents didn't find it as funny as we did."

"Exactly. Now try to remember the evening. Who were you able to talk to that night?"

"Well, Grandmother Terra was next to me, so I could talk to her. On my other side was my cousin, so I talked to them too. So, the two people I talked to that night were my cousin and Grandmother Terra, the two people who I was sitting next to at the table."

"Yes. Well, the channels are the same way. They can talk to the channel that sits next to them on the channel clock. So, for example, let's look at this image.

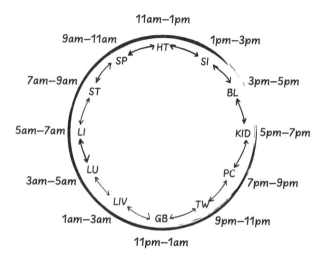

"Here we can see that:

HT interacts with SP and SI

SI interacts with HT and BL

BL interacts with SI and KID

KID interacts with BL and PC

PC interacts with KID and TW

TW interacts with PC and GB

GB interacts with TW and LIV

LIV interacts with GB and LU

LU interacts with LIV and LI

LI interacts with LU and ST

ST interacts with LI and SP

SP interacts with ST and HT.

"And that brings us back to HT."

"Easy enough. I will have to remember the new codes for the channels based on the abbreviations of the organ names. But I get the idea. Any channel that is before or after another channel can interact with those channels."

"Yes, that is true. Now look closely at the clock and the interactions. Do you notice anything?"

"I notice lots of things. But I think I know what you are going to say. We saw a lot of these interactions yesterday. For example, Hand Shao Yin Heart interacts with Hand Tai Yang Small Intestine in System 1 Interior/Exterior already. Also, Hand Tai Yang Small Intestine interacts with Foot Tai Yang Bladder in System 2 Full Channels, and here in this system."

"That is what we were hoping you would notice—that each channel will have two interactions if we look at the clock. One of those two interactions will always be the same as System 1 Interior/Exterior. This is because we used this system to place the channels, if you remember, so it is logical that they are always next to each other. So, in order to make things simple, we will now add another rule for System 4 Biorhythm Neighbors. Only channels that are next to each other and have the same Yin-Yang polarity will be part of System 4. So, an example is:

> Hand Shao Yin Heart is between 11am and 1pm. The channels that come before and after it are Foot Tai Yin Spleen and Hand Tai Yang Small Intestine. Hand Shao Yin Heart and Foot Tai Yin Spleen are both Yin, so they will interact with each other in System 4 Biorhythm Neighbors.

"And this is true for all the other channels. So we would say:

Hand Shao Yin Heart interacts with Foot Tai Yin Spleen

Hand Tai Yang Small Intestine interacts with Foot Tai Yang Bladder

Foot Shao Yin Kidney interacts with Hand Jue Yin Pericardium

Hand Shao Yang Triple Warmer interacts with Foot Shao Yang Gall Bladder

Foot Jue Yin Liver interacts with Hand Tai Yin Lung

Hand Yang Ming Large Intestine interacts with Foot Yang Ming Stomach."

Sun listened and then added, "So, for the Yin channels, there is a new relationship here. But for the Yang channels, it is the same as System 2 Full Channels."

"Yes. Systems 2 Full Channels and 4 Biorhythm Neighbors are the same for all the Yang channels. And when we think about how the clock was created and we used the Yang channels to describe the movements of the sun, it makes sense.

"A good way to think about it is to imagine the old story of King Arthur and the Knights of the Round Table. But instead of medieval knights, we will have the channels of the body and the round table. So, let's imagine that the Yang channels are the knights and the Yin channels are the maidens or wives of the knights."

Both Sun and Grandfather Terra gave Grandmother Terra a weird look. She replied, "I know that this is old fashioned and that anyone could be a knight and it doesn't matter if it is male or female, but for this analogy it is helpful, so please indulge me.

"So, we have the Channel Knights of the Round Clock. As dictated by tradition, each pair of Yin and Yang must sit next to each other at the table. So, Heart will be next to Small Intestine, and so on. Now, as these are feudal times and we cannot trust Yin channels to talk to Yang channels that they are not in an Interior/Exterior relationship with, on the other side of the channels that aren't their System 1 Interior/Exterior partner we will put the same polarity of channel. So, Yin will be next to Yin, and Yang will be next to Yang. The Yin channels, which in our analogy are the females or stay at the castle channels, will have time to talk with each other and exchange on how their castles and projects at home are doing. The Yang channels, which are the traveling knights, will be able to reminisce about their exploits as knights of the realm. And they will have their Yin-Yang partner on the other side of them. It is just an image to help understand the system.

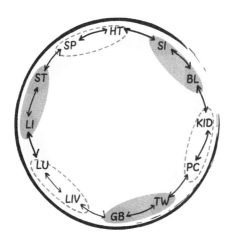

For Yin channels, these are new interactions.	*Same as System 2* Full Channels for Yang channels. Included in System 4.	*Same as System 1* Interior/Exterior. Not included in System 4.

"And if we were to look at the same pattern in the UAT model just to see, it would look like this image."

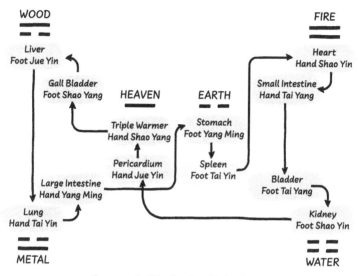

System 4: Biorhythm Neighbors

Sun looked at the UAT model. "It reminds me of a figure eight on its side. It's as if it never ends. And I see that the new relationships are when it goes from one element to another element."

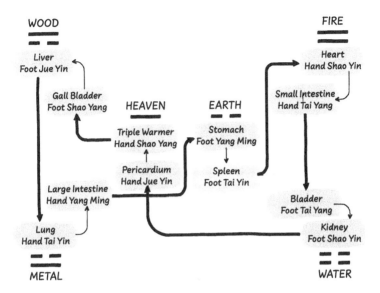

"Great. Now let's try using it. But first, if we were to treat someone with System 4 Biorhythm Neighbors, would we treat them on the same side as the problem or the other side?"

Sun thought and then answered, "This system is based on both channels having the same polarity. Both are either Yin or Yang. So, as they have the same Yin-Yang polarity, they must always be treated opposite side."

"So, let's treat someone. A person has pain in the chest area, very close to the bone in the middle of the chest, just in the space where the ribs meet the sternum. It is at about the same area as the nipple, on the left side. First job, what is the affected channel?"

"Well, it is close to the midline of the front, which in a weird way actually is a channel that is associated with the back of the body. I remember that from last year. It is at the nipple but the channel continues below the diaphragm, so it is a foot channel. And it is Yin. So, it is the Foot Yin channel of the back or Foot Shao Yin Kidney."

"Yes. And now, based on System 4 Biorhythm Neighbors, what channel interacts with Foot Shao Yin Kidney?"

Sun looked at the clock diagram. "Foot Shao Yin Kidney is between 5pm and 7pm. The channels that surround it are the Foot Tai Yang Bladder and the Hand Jue Yin Pericardium. The one that has the same polarity as the Foot Shao Yin Kidney is the Hand Jue Yin Pericardium. So that is the channel I would use."

"Very good. Now the pain is on the left side, which side would you treat?"

"This is a foot channel interacting with a hand channel, so they have one polarity, but they are two Yin channels, so they do not have that polarity. So, I would treat opposite side, right side."

"And where would you look for points on the right Hand Jue Yin Pericardium channel to image the problem at the sixth intercostal space on the Foot Shao Yin Kidney channels?"

"Hmm. I would use the image of the hand is the head, the wrist is the neck, and the forearm is from the collar bone to the navel. And that would be in the upper area closer to the wrist. I could turn the image around and use the muscle in the upper arm."

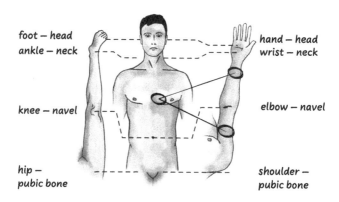

foot – head
ankle – neck

hand – head
wrist – neck

knee – navel

elbow – navel

hip –
pubic bone

shoulder –
pubic bone

"That is excellent, Sun. You have followed all the steps and found the treatments. What is interesting about this example is that the images on the Hand Jue Yin Pericardium channel that have both of the points that are in these areas—Tainquan PC 2 for the upper arm and Jianshi PC 5 and Neiquan PC 6—are all indicated for heart pain and palpitations. And the Foot Shao Yin Kidney goes over the Heart organ itself. So you see, by using this idea we are able to find the points that the acupuncture books say treat a particular problem, and we can get there with logic and reasoning and not just memorizing all the points and the actions."

"I see. So, now that I understand this logic, I know everything in acupuncture?"

"Well, that is maybe going a bit far. There are still other theories and things to add. But it will help a lot and explains most of the distal actions of the points we find in the texts."

"OK. So now there is only one more time system to study. First, more tea, please."

CHAPTER 17

DANCING PARTNERS

System 5: Biorhythm Opposites

Grandfather Terra poured Sun another cup of tea. Grandmother Terra started again. "So, you want the last time-based system, do you? Well, OK. This one is called Biorhythm Opposites or sometimes it is referred to as the Law of Midday/Midnight. Let's go back to the Chinese meal last year where we tried to make shrimp fly. I was on one side of you and your cousin was on the other side of you, so that is who you talked with the whole evening. Was there anyone else you communicated with that evening, but without talking?"

"I was making funny faces with Grandfather Terra who was sitting across from me. He kept trying to make me laugh but didn't really succeed until he was helping us speed up the middle turning thing and make it go really fast. The restaurant scolded him but let us off. That is what made me laugh, so I communicated with the person directly opposite me."

"Excellent, Sun! We got into a lot of trouble with your parents after that night. They said we were bad influences on you. We will leave that for another time. Anyway, just as you communicated with the person directly across from you at the table, the channel can interact directly with the channels directly across from it on the clock.

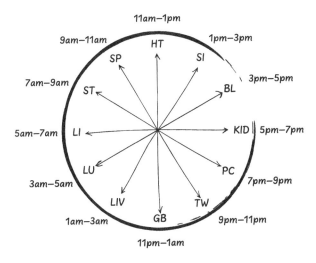

"Now we can also use our story before of the knights and the maidens. As we saw in System 4, the Yang channel knights are either sitting next to their Yin partner (the maiden) or their fellow Yang knight who they go out on adventures with. It would be unseemly for them to be seen talking to another maiden that they were not in a System 1 Interior/Exterior relationship with. However, they can look. And each Yang channel knight when they look across the table finds a beautiful maiden in the form of a Yin channel. And every Yin channel maiden when they look across the table sees a handsome knight in the form of a Yang channel. And even more than that, the opposite Yin or Yang channel that is across from them is even more exotic because they are also on an opposite limb. Now, Sun, you are a little young yet to have romantic feelings, or maybe you are not. Anyway, to have a beautiful maiden from a distant limb sitting across from you can be acceptable but it would never be OK to sit next to one. So, in this story, across from every Hand Yang channel sits a Yin Foot channel, and across from every Foot Yang channel sits a Hand Yin channel."

Grandfather Terra laughed. "I think your grandmother misses reading you fairy tales. But it is a good analogy of understanding System 5 Biorhythm Opposites or Midday/Midnight. I will show you another way to think about this relationship. We can imagine every channel as a wave function. It will have a high point, zenith, and a low point, nadir. For example, look at the Hand Shao Yin Heart channel.

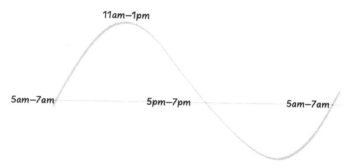

Qi in Hand Shao Yin Heart channel seen as a wave function

"Now this is true for every channel. They will all have the same function, but the times of the zenith and the nadir will change. So, another channel will have the same image but the times will change. Like the Foot Shao Yang Gall Bladder channel.

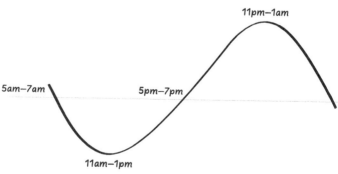

Qi in Foot Shao Yang Gall Bladder channel seen as a wave function

"We will see here that just the times of the zenith and the nadir changed. Or we could also use the terms 'peak' for the high point and 'trough' for the low point. This is what is used for waves in the ocean. Now when we put the Hand Shao Yin Heart and the Foot Shao Yang Gall Bladder channels together, we see the following:

Qi in Hand Shao Yin Heart channel seen as a wave function with the Foot Shao Yang Gall Bladder as a wave function

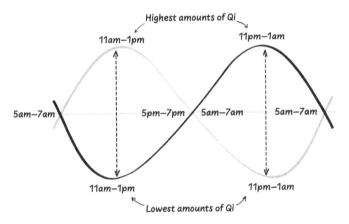

"We see that the Hand Shao Yin Heart has its peak at the same time as the Foot Shao Yang Gall Bladder has its trough, and vice versa."

Grandmother Terra interjected, "It's as if they are dancing after dinner. When one channel steps forward, the other steps back. When one channel steps right, the other steps left. They are in perfect unison in their movements, although their movements are the exact opposites of each other."

Sun nodded. "I think you miss socializing, Grandmother. I see what you are saying. It is as if they are in perfect unison yet completely opposite. What does this system look like on the UAT model?"

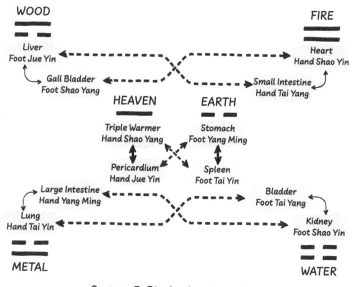

System 5: Biorhythm Opposites

Grandfather Terra showed Sun. "It looks like three separate horizontal figure eights when we add System 1 to it. If we use Grandmother Terra's idea of the dinner table, in System 4 Biorhythm Neighbors, if one channel wants to send a message to another channel across from it, it needs to send the information through all the channels that are between it and the other channel. It is like the game Telephone. In System 5 Biorhythm Opposites, it is a shortcut across the table."

"I liked playing Telephone. It is always funny to see how the message almost never stays the same at the end. So, I guess that this system has a balancing effect to that. It helps channels that are so far apart from each other communicate."

"That is a great analogy, Sun. This system, and the last system, transmit information quickly that would normally be difficult to communicate, and so it gets fast results. It might take longer for the results to solidify and more treatments might be needed, but it will get the results very quickly.

"Now let's put it into practice. A patient has pain on the side of the neck and a headache that is on the side of the head. What would you do? Remember to do all the steps in order."

"First, I would identify the problem channel. As it is the side of the neck and the head, I would say the side channels are the problem. As it is in the neck and the head, it would be a Yang channel. And as the pain is above the eyes, it would be a foot channel. So, the foot side Yang channel is the Foot Shao Yang Gall Bladder. As we saw, the Foot Shao Yang Gall Bladder is opposite the Hand Shao Yin Heart channel on the clock, so I would use the hand Shao Yin Heart to treat.

"I think the best image is the arm and hand together because the wrist can be the neck and the hand the head."

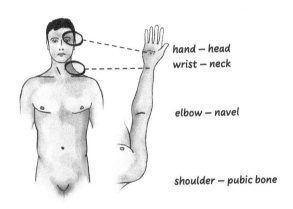

hand – head
wrist – neck

elbow – navel

shoulder – pubic bone

"You have got it all, Sun. We would put the needles from the wrist and up into the hand. If we used the acupuncture points as a reference, we would put needles from Tongli HT 5 to Shaofu HT 8. We could put five to seven needles along the Hand Shao Yin Heart channel here. And as this system has a Foot Yang channel interacting with a Hand Yin channel, there are already the two basic polarities, so it can be used on either side."

Sun was happy. "I get it. For the time similarity there are two systems: System 4 Biorhythm Neighbors and System 5 Biorhythm Opposites. System 4 uses the channel that is next to it and has the same polarity on the biorhythm clock. System 5 uses the channel that is directly opposite and has a complementary and opposite wave function to it. System 4 has to be opposite side because the channels change limbs but have the same Yin-Yang polarity, and System 5 can be either side because the channels interacting are both opposite limb and opposite Yin-Yang polarity. Also, for System 4, the Yang channel relationships are the same as System 2 Full Channels. And now after drinking all this tea, I think I need to use the bathroom."

Exposure to Sunlight-Based Channel Interactions

CHAPTER 18

WHAT IS IN A NAME?

System 6: Exposure to Sunlight

The last few days had been a whirlwind of ideas and newness. Sun realized that their grandparents had been taking their time with all the basic information and theory and were now moving ahead and sharing much more. This made sense, as Sun knew their time with the grandparents was quickly winding down. In a few days, Sun would have to go back to their normal life. They called that life the normal, boring life, and when they were with their grandparents, it was the real life—real in that Sun felt more like themselves, whatever that meant, and they felt they were alive. Sun knew that this feeling would not last when they went back to their normal life, yet this year Sun felt more comfortable about returning because they felt they had more tools to cope with their difficult emotions. They had the Qi Gong exercises to help move their Qi or energy, they understood more about how their emotions were signals for a response to something, and they were learning how to feel and express what was happening in their body. It would still be difficult, but they felt more ready than before.

Sun was explaining this to Grandfather Terra as they were doing some gardening. Grandfather Terra was nodding his head and smiling. "Sun, that is a very honest assessment.

You are aware of the challenges that you face and the tools that you have. You are also aware of what you still need to work on. And being honest with where we are, and able to look at life from this place, is a key life skill. The more honest we are with ourselves, the more honest we can be with others. Most people tell more lies to themselves than to the outside world. This is not because they are doing it on purpose. It is a way of protecting themselves. People think they need to feel strong about themselves to face the world. They think that if they show weakness that other people will take advantage of them or hurt them. That it can be an illusion, meaning that it seems true, but once you get beyond the surface of the idea, it does not hold up anymore. Real strength comes from being honest with yourself about what and who you are, and engaging in working with even the most difficult parts of yourself."

Sun thought they understood but wanted to make sure. "Could you give me an example of how you are honest with yourself, and work with it?"

Grandfather Terra shook his head, laughed, and blushed all at the same time. "The perfect question to throw my words back at me. Very well, I will give you an example about myself. As you know, I am married to one of the most brilliant people I have ever known—your grandmother. Not only is she very smart intellectually, but she is also very aware of her emotions and what is happening. When she gives her opinion, most of the time she will be proved correct. She also reads people very well. She is able to understand not only how they will behave, but also why they are behaving in the way they do. And when I hear her talk, I have many different emotions and feelings that all seem to contradict each other and yet are all there at the same time.

"A part of me fills with pride and inspiration. I am proud that someone so wonderful has chosen to spend their life with me, and I am inspired to continue to learn more about the world and myself. Another part of me feels insignificant and not up to the task of being her equal. This is a heavier feeling, and it usually shows up in my abdomen. It is linked to me not appreciating my own worth and value. It is an old voice that has been there since I was younger than you are now. There are also other feelings that pile on. I can have some anger that she is always the star, and I am second fiddle. I sometimes also feel honored to be her contemporary. I can feel a competitive side to myself that I do not really like. And so on. I have all these emotions and I am discovering new ones every day, even after being with her for over 40 years.

"Now, I am honest about how I feel and what is happening inside when it happens. I write about it, talk about it with my close friends, and also share it with your grandmother. And the more honest I am, especially about the more difficult emotions, to myself and others, the more I learn about myself. Those emotions do not just go away, they become part of my conscious, daily life and are not these heavy things that I carry around my neck. What is very curious is that the more I am open and honest about them, the more they show themselves. And the more they show themselves, the easier they are to accept and understand. They are just aspects, like all the other aspects of myself, that make me a person. I also understand my own behaviors more, too. You and your grandmother love making fun of me when I go into lecture mode. And I love you both for it because it reminds me that lecture mode is often linked to me feeling less important, so I make myself more important. That I have people who remind me that I do not have to be important to be loved is a great gift."

"Wow. I was not expecting all of that. I never realized that you could also feel different or have problems with your emotions and dealing with people. I always imagined you as perfect. Well, now I only have Grandmother Terra as the only perfect one left."

"Very funny, Sun, and perhaps a little true."

When it got to teatime, Sun was ready for the last system. The system about the sun. This was their system. "So, can you tell me how I have become a system of channel interactions?" asked Sun.

Grandmother Terra smiled. "How did you become a system of channel interactions? I remember that the last system we will look at is based on the sun. More precisely, how much sunlight each channel gets in relation to the other channels. Let's take a look. First, we will just remember the basics. There are two main types of channels, Yin and Yang. And how do we identify if the channel is Yin or Yang?"

"By how much sunlight they get. The body has the Yang part, which is on the back, the head, and the exterior parts of the limbs. The other part, the Yin, is on the torso, although there are some Yang channels there too, and the interior parts of the limbs. The Yang gets more sunlight than the Yin."

"Excellent, Sun. And now on each aspect of the body there is a Yin and a Yang part, except for the head which is only Yang. But as we are using the limbs to understand the channel interactions, we can forget about that. And now that we have these two pain aspects, Yin and Yang, we also divide the body into three segments on each aspect: front, middle, and back."

"Yes, I know all this," said Sun. "There are:

Yin front

Yang front

Yin middle

Yang middle

Yin back

Yang back.

"We have gone over this many times."

"True. Now do you remember what the Chinese names for these channels are?"

"Yin front is Tai Yin

Yin middle is Jue Yin

Yin back is Shao Yin

Yang front is Yang Ming

Yang middle is Shao Yang

Yang back is Tai Yang."

"Good, now what do those names refer to?"

"The Yin or Yang in the name is if the channel is on the Yin or Yang aspect of the body. The other words refer to how much sunlight that aspect of the body gets:

Tai: most amount of sunlight

Shao: least amount of sunlight

Jue or Ming: medium amount of sunlight."

"You are an excellent student as always, Sun. So, it would look like the following."

Amount of Sunlight Exposure

Amount of Sunlight	Yang channels	Yin channels
Most	Tai Yang	Tai Yin
Medium	Yang Ming	Jue Yin
Least	Shao Yang	Shao Yin

"OK. I remember all this from every other conversation we

have had on channels. What I want to know is how this creates a system of the channel interactions."

Grandfather Terra coughed. "Sun, we know you can get impatient, but please remember that we have a reason for repeating everything so often. It helps you to understand and hold on to the information and use it better. Now the answer to your question is quite simple. A Yang channel that gets a certain amount of sun in relationship to the other Yang channels will interact with a Yin channel that gets a certain amount of sun in relationship to the other Yin channels. So, this means that:

Most sun on Yang interacts with most sun on Yin

Medium sun on Yang interacts with medium sun on Yin

Least sun on Yang interacts with least sun on Yin.

"Or:

Tai Yang interacts with Tai Yin

Yang Ming interacts with Jue Yin

Shao Yang interacts with Shao Yin."

"Yes, I know that you have a reason for it. Just sometimes I want to move forward so much it is difficult. I guess that is one of those things I can be more honest about with myself—the feeling that I understand something quicker than most other people. So, is that the whole system?"

"Not quite. There is one other aspect: it only works between a hand channel and a foot channel. So, the full idea is:

Hand Tai Yang interacts with Foot Tai Yin

Hand Yang Ming interacts with Foot Jue Yin

Hand Shao Yang interacts with Foot Shao Yin

Foot Tai Yang interacts with Hand Tai Yin

Foot Yang Ming interacts with Hand Jue Yin

Foot Shao Yang interacts with Hand Shao Yin.

"Or:

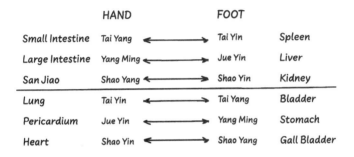

	HAND			FOOT	
Small Intestine	Tai Yang	←	→	Tai Yin	Spleen
Large Intestine	Yang Ming	←	→	Jue Yin	Liver
San Jiao	Shao Yang	←	→	Shao Yin	Kidney
Lung	Tai Yin	←	→	Tai Yang	Bladder
Pericardium	Jue Yin	←	→	Yang Ming	Stomach
Heart	Shao Yin	←	→	Shao Yang	Gall Bladder

"This is called System 6 Exposure to Sunlight. The name is saying that we are using one channel on the arm and one channel on the leg that get the same amount of sunlight and have opposite Yin-Yang polarities."

"OK, I get it. That is why it is so important to understand the Chinese names of the channels, as it is the basis of this system. Also, your definition of the system stated that there is a hand channel interacting with a foot channel and a Yin channel interacting with a Yang channel. Does that mean that both base polarities have been met and it can be used on either side?"

"Very perceptive, Sun. Yes, that is exactly what it means. Now this system when put on the UAT model gives an interesting image. Take a look.

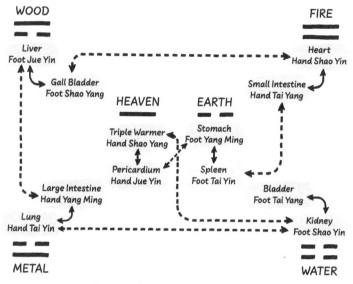

System 6: Exposure to Sunlight

"Do you see how it makes a loop in the center where there is heaven and earth and then goes out to the fire and water and then connects wood and metal? It makes an image like this:

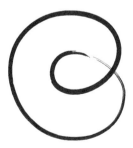

"Have you ever seen an image like this before?"

Sun followed the image with their finger and thought. "Yes, I have. In biology class. That is what a cell looks like just before it divides into two. What was the name for that process again?"

"It is called mitosis. And you are correct. It is the image of cell division. In fact, this system is extremely interesting. But first, let's finish understanding it in relation to the channel interactions before that.

"When you look at it on the UAT model and compare it to System 5 Biorhythm Opposites, do you notice anything?"

Sun looked at both images side by side.

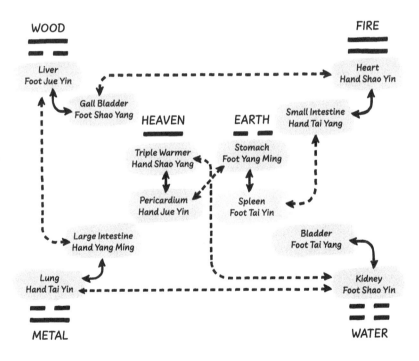

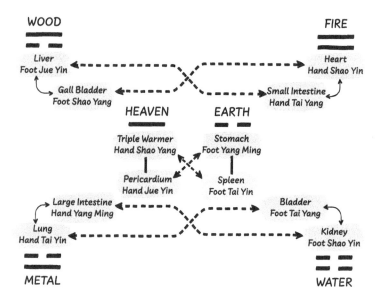

"There are some of the same interactions. In fact, it is the interactions that are horizontal that are the same."

"Yes. The horizontal interactions are the same. This is when a Yin Hand channel is interacting with a Yang Foot channel. The vertical interactions are between a Yin Foot and a Yang Hand, and these are new interactions. So, we can say that Systems 5 and 6 are the same for the Hand Yin and the Foot Leg channels.

"Now let's put this to use. A person has pain directly on their nipple on the left side. Walk me through the process of treatment."

Sun sat up.

"Step 1: Identify the affected channel. In this case it is the Foot Yang Ming Stomach.

Step 2: Establish which channel interacts with the affected channel. If we use System 6 Exposure to Sunlight,

Foot Yang Ming gets the medium amount of sunlight on the Yang side of the foot. The channel that gets the same, medium amount of sunlight, but is on the opposite Yin-Yang side and limb, is the Hand Jue Yin Pericardium.

Step 3: Image the affected area onto the interaction channel. In this case, I would use the image of the forearm or the upper arm."

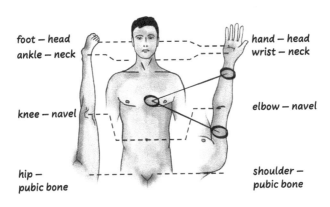

foot – head
ankle – neck

hand – head
wrist – neck

knee – navel

elbow – navel

hip –
pubic bone

shoulder –
pubic bone

Sun looked at the image and then said, "Hang on a minute. This was the same image and the same treatment we did for the problem on the Foot Shao Yin Kidney channel for System 4. In this case, we are treating the Foot Yang Ming Stomach with the Hand Jue Yin Pericardium and using the points in the forearm or the upper arm, but it is the exact same treatment."

"Very good, Sun. So here we are concentrating on the Foot Yang Ming Stomach channel which interacts with Hand Jue Yin Pericardium. And we find that the treatment is the same for a problem in the same area on the Foot Shao Yin Kidney, as the Hand Jue Yin Pericardium interacts with both channels. In this area is the Heart organ which both the

Foot Shao Yin Kidney and the Foot Yang Ming Stomach pass through. And we understand why the acupuncture manuals say that points on the Hand Jue Yin Pericardium channel in these areas treat the Heart organ problems. Because of channel interactions and imaging and mirroring."

"Wow! That is amazing. We found the points without memorizing them, but they just appeared out of the logic of the channel interactions. That is awesome. What was the interesting point you wanted to make about this system, Grandfather Terra?"

"Well, I am glad you asked. We were talking about the image of cell division. Well, that image is also like a horizontal figure eight lying on its side. But instead of the two loops next to each other, one is inside the other. And the middle circle or center has the elements heaven and earth. In Chinese philosophy, heaven and earth are the first separation of Yin and Yang. They are the beginning of all things, and here they are at the center of the system.

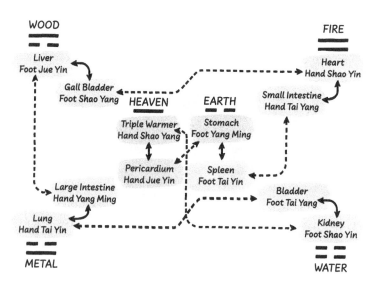

"Then the two elements that interact with heaven and earth are fire and water.

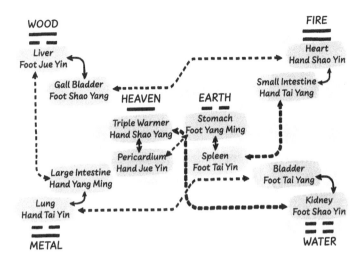

"Earth interacts with fire, and heaven with water. So, the original Yang (heaven) interacts with the most Yin (water), and the original Yin (earth) interacts with the most Yang (fire). Fire and water are born from heaven and earth. Heaven and earth are these big ideas, but we can't really hold them or touch them. Yes, we can touch the soil and rock, but the earth as a whole planet is too vast to imagine holding. We cannot hold fire and water either but can see them and work with them. We are moving from the subtle to the less subtle.

"From fire and water, we move into the even less subtle realm, into the elements of wood and metal. Again, Yang will interact with Yin, fire interacting with wood, and Yin will interact with Yang, water interacting with metal.

"And then fire will interact with wood and water with metal.

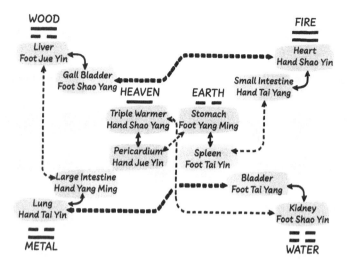

"Wood and metal are both mixed elements as they have both a Yin and a Yang line in their image. Wood is Yin with a manifestation of Yang, and metal is Yang with a manifestation of Yin. This is Chinese philosophy, when the 10,000 myriad things come into existence. It is the manifestation of life. Wood and metal are both elements that we can hold and manipulate. We can change their shape and create tools from them. They represent the material, everyday world.

"So, we have the three levels of manifestation:

The first level of heaven and earth, too vast to really comprehend.

The second level of fire and water, which we can see but not hold.

The third level of metal and wood, which is the most manifest, and we can not only hold but also manipulate.

"System 6 Exposure to Sunlight is a microcosm of how Yin and Yang interact and mutually create each other."

Sun was taken a bit aback. They were not expecting that. "I had no idea that the systems could also be used to understand anything else but channels. This is amazing."

Grandmother Terra smiled. "Yes, your grandfather is brilliant when he talks about his passion. He always says that I am the brilliant one, but as we both know that is just those parts of him that hold his difficult emotion. He is truly very intelligent and wise."

Sun nodded. "Well, at least he lets his difficult emotions talk. And yes, a very wise, smart person indeed."

Grandfather Terra laughed. "Thank you both. And now I think all of us can benefit from the wisdom of a nice dinner."

PUTTING IT INTO PRACTICE

CHAPTER 19

A FAMILY MATTER

A Look at All Six Systems Together

Another day passed in the lives of Sun and the Grandparents Terra. They felt happy to be spending time with each other and a sadness was creeping in that their summer together was coming to an end. Sun would have to go home soon, and all their lives would return to their normal patterns, but not really. During an afternoon walk Sun began talking. "It will be strange going back to my parents and school life. This happens every year at the same time. I return home and find that the summer feels as if it was a dream, as if it happened, but not really. Thank you for the book you gave me last year, it really helped me remember that it wasn't a dream. I would sometimes look at it and I would forget about the channels and remember our walks and discussions. It wasn't the contents of the discussions that were what I remembered, but what you were wearing at the time, or the sounds of the birds, or something about the environment. And those memories gave me a nice warm feeling."

Grandfather Terra put his hand on Sun's shoulder and communicated his love with a gentle squeeze. "We will miss you too, Sun. We really enjoy having you visit us. In fact, your grandmother and I have been talking and we think we will start teaching more again. You have reignited our love for sharing our knowledge, and for that we owe you a great thank you. So, thank you, Sun."

"Will this mean that you will be traveling more and be in my hometown where the school you taught at is?"

"That is what it looks like, Sun. So, this coming year you should be seeing more of us than before. And we hope you will perhaps come to visit us at the school sometimes."

"I would love that. And I guess if I will be visiting you at the school, I better really understand all the channels and their interactions, so I can help you with your teaching." Sun had a mischievous look in their eye as they said the last words.

Grandmother Terra laughed. "Exactly, Sun. We will almost definitely need an assistant. And there is no one better than you for that job."

Sun felt a huge weight lift inside them. They would get to see their grandparents much more this year. And they would be teaching acupuncture again. Sun's mind was racing with a 1000 questions, and one stood out the most. "So, if I will be your assistant, I guess you better really show me how all this works together. I mean, I can see each system individually, but I would like to get a big picture of all the systems together."

Grandfather Terra shook his head and grinned. "Always ready to keep that mind of yours moving. Alright, let's have a seat and try to paint a full picture. First let's go over some of the basics. How many systems are there?"

"There are six systems."

"And what is the basis of the systems?"

"There are three types of similarities:

Space

Time

Exposure to sunlight."

"And how many systems are in each type?"

"There are:

Three based on space

Two based on time

One based on exposure to sunlight."

"Very good, Sun. Now let's try creating a story about all the systems to see if we can find how they fit together. And I think using Grandmother Terra's analogy of the Knights of the Round Table is a good start. Let's start with the systems based on space. As space is the physical one of the systems, we will use it for the base. Now, how about we imagine that System 1 Interior/Exterior is like a married couple? We can say that the Yin channel is the female partner, and the Yang channel is the male partner. Together they live in the same house, which we will call the element. So:

In the house of metal live Hand Tai Yin Lung and Hand Yang Ming Large Intestine.

In the house of earth live Foot Tai Yin Spleen and Foot Yang Ming Stomach.

In the house of heaven live Hand Jue Yin Liver and Hand Shao Yang Triple Warmer.

In the house of wood live Foot Jue Yin Liver and Foot Shao Yang Gall Bladder.

In the house of fire live Hand Shao Yin Heart and Foot Tai Yang Small Intestine.

In the house of water live Foot Shao Yin Kidney and Foot Tai Yang Bladder."

Sun responded, "OK, I see that. So, System 1 is like a married couple. How about System 2?"

"System 2 Full Channels we will associate with brothers and sisters. Let's assume that the channels live in a land where they do not change their names but keep their names of their parents when they get married. We will say that the full names of the channels are the family names. So, the channels would mean that:

Hand Tai Yin Lung and Foot Tai Yin Spleen are sisters.

Hand Jue Yin Pericardium and Foot Jue Yin Liver are sisters.

Hand Shao Yin Heart and Foot Shao Yin Kidney are sisters.

Hand Yang Ming Large Intestine and Foot Yang Ming Stomach are brothers.

Hand Shao Yang Triple Warmer and Foot Shao Yang Gall Bladder are brothers.

Hand Tai Yang Small Intestine and Foot Tai Yang Bladder are brothers.

"System 2 Full Channels is about sibling relationships."

"I think I see where this is going. System 1 is about married couples, System 2 is about brothers and sisters. Now System 3 Closed Circuit Channels would be…hmm. I know, brothers and sisters-in-law."

Grandmother Terra raised her eyebrows. "Brothers and sisters-in-law?"

Sun sat up. "Well, let's take the Hand Tai Yin channel. The Hand Tai Yin channel is married to the Hand Yang Ming Large Intestine. That is System 1. The Hand Tai Yin channel's sister is the Foot Tai Yin Spleen. That is System 2.

"Hand Yang Ming Large Intestine's brother is Foot Yang Ming Stomach, and Foot Yang Ming Stomach is married to Foot Tai Yin Spleen. So, System 3 Closed Circuit Channels is the relationship between Hand Tai Yin Lung and Foot Yang Ming Stomach. So, they have an in-law relationship. And I guess this means that both brothers from the same family married both sisters from another family. Let's say that the channels live in a weird world where that is the only way it can happen."

"Brilliant, Sun. I love it! So, we have three family relationships so far:

System 1 Interior/Exterior: Married couples

System 2 Full Channels: Brothers and sisters

System 3 Closed Circuit Channels: Brothers-in-law and sisters-in-law.

"Now what about the time systems?"

Sun was enjoying using their imagination to explain the channels. "Well, I think we should use your image from the other day of the round table. In the Realm of Channels there are six important houses, which are the six elements. And these six houses like to get together often for dinner. When they get together, they sit around a big round table. As it is an important meal, they all have specific places they have to sit. We talked about why they sit there when we talked about the clock. As they always sit in the same places, we can say they have dining partners. System 4 is Biorhythm Neighbors. Or now it is same polarity dining partners. And System 5 Biorhythm Opposites is opposite polarity googly-eyed partners."

"Googly-eyed? Why googly-eyed?" questioned Grandfather Terra.

"Because they make googly eyes at each other across the table. They cannot talk but they can look at each other and make googly eyes."

"Very well. System 5 Biorhythm Opposites is googly-eyed pairs. Now how about System 6 Exposure to Sunlight, how does that fit into our story?"

Sun was thinking. "I know. System 6 is about cousins. In System 6 Exposure to Sunlight, we use only part of the Chinese name. We use the Tai, Shao, or Ming and Jue. If the two channels have the same name, then they are cousins. And for the Ming and the Jue, they used to have the same family name but the Jue part of the family changed their name because of a rivalry between the two families a long time ago. And now the two families are back together but they still keep their new names. Also, this system of cousins only uses opposite limbs and polarities, because of the Ming and Jue feud. So a Hand Jue Yin and Foot Yang Ming can talk because they are not a threat to each other. But when a Hand Jue Yin and Hand Yang Ming talk, there is still a rivalry, so they cannot interact."

"Very inventive, Sun. So, let's recap the story:

There is a Realm of Channels. In this Realm of Channels there are six main houses, and each house has the name of an element. In each element lives a married couple that share the same position on the same limb. This is System 1 Interior/Exterior.

Each of the partners of an element has either a brother or sister that lives in the same position but on a different limb. They share the same full channel name with their siblings. This is System 2 Full Channels.

In this realm, both siblings find their partners in other pairs that are siblings. So their brother's wife is also their wife's sister (that is very complicated to say in a simple sentence). This is System 3 Closed Circuit Channels.

Now in this realm, the six main houses love to have feasts, and at their feasts they all sit around a big, circular table. When they are sitting at the table, it is the Yang channels that decide where they sit, and they always want to sit next to their brother on one side (System 2) and their partner on the other side (System 1). This means that the Yin channels are sitting next to their partners on one side and they find themselves next to another Yin channel on their left. This Yin channel is not their sister but a new channel they can interact with. This is System 4 Biorhythm Neighbors.

During these meals, the channels like to have a merry time telling stories and laughing with the channels sitting next to them. As they are in a happy mood, they tend to notice others in a happy mood. And sitting directly across from them is always a channel from another limb and a different polarity. This beautiful, exotic channel sitting directly opposite them likes to make googly eyes at them and they can communicate that way. This is System 5 Biorhythm Opposites.

Now the Realm of Channels has a long history and there have been big feuds between the different families. One time, the feud was not between families but within the family. The Family of Ming had such a difficult past that they split into two families, the Ming and the Jue. But now, after a long period, they can tolerate each other and have started to talk to each other again. However, when it comes to the distant cousin relationships there is a special bond that happens when there are absolute polarities. This means both the opposite limb and the opposite hand polarity. When cousins who have this relationship meet, they have a strong interaction we call System 6 Exposure to Sunlight.

"How is that, Sun?"

"I love it. It is a real story and I feel as if the channels come to life. OK. Now I have another question."

Grandfather Terra held up his hand. "First, let's get the tea ready and then we will continue."

CHAPTER 20

GETTING TO THE POINT

Shortcuts and How to Choose Images

With tea on the table and in their cups, Sun started again. "As I was saying, I have another question. We have looked at the six systems of how the channels interact, and that means that each channel can have up to six interactions. On top of that there are many different images that exist. How do I know which channel interaction to use and which image?"

Grandmother Terra nodded. "That is the million-dollar question that is always asked when we teach this course. There are a few ways we can answer the question. The first is that all of the systems work and all of the images work. So even if you do not choose the 'most indicated' channel and image you will still get a result. And the easiest way to choose is through palpation. This means that you take all the channels that interact with the problem area and all the images. You then palpate all of these interacting channels with their images and treat the most sensitive points, or Achi points in Chinese. When we teach in schools, this is often where we start as it is a good practice for a beginner in this method.

"So, let's look at a simple example. A person has pain in the left ankle on the Foot Jue Yin Liver channel area. Our first step is the diagnosis. This is Foot Jue Yin Liver at the ankle. The next step is to identify the interaction channels."

"OK. Let me go through them. The first three systems are based on space. The Foot Jue Yin Liver is in the middle of the leg on the Yin part of the foot. So, all other middle channels will interact with it—or all its immediate family of husband, sister, and brother-in-law will interact with it:

System 1: Foot Shao Yang Gall Bladder

System 2: Hand Jue Yin Pericardium

System 3: Hand Shao Yang Triple Warmer.

"The next two systems are based on time—the channel sitting next to it with the same polarity and the channel sitting opposite it with a different polarity and on a different limb:

System 4: Hand Tai Yin Lung

System 5: Hand Tai Yang Small Intestine.

"The last system is based on the sun—the channel on the opposite limb and polarity that gets the relative same amount of sun:

System 6: Hand Yang Ming Large Intestine."

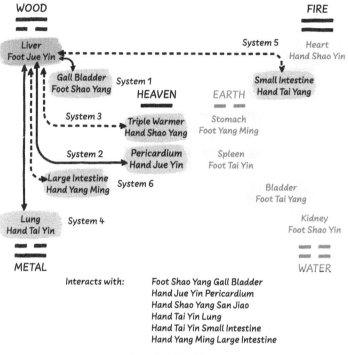

WOOD

Liver
Foot Jue Yin

Gall Bladder
Foot Shao Yang   System 1
               HEAVEN

System 3   Triple Warmer
           Hand Shao Yang

System 2   Pericardium
           Hand Jue Yin

Large Intestine
Hand Yang Ming   System 6

Lung   System 4
Hand Tai Yin

METAL

FIRE

System 5   Heart
           Hand Shao Yin

Small Intestine
Hand Tai Yang

EARTH   Stomach
        Foot Yang Ming

Spleen
Foot Tai Yin

Bladder
Foot Tai Yang

Kidney
Foot Shao Yin

WATER

Interacts with: Foot Shao Yang Gall Bladder
                  Hand Jue Yin Pericardium
                  Hand Shao Yang San Jiao
                  Hand Tai Yin Lung
                  Hand Tai Yin Small Intestine
                  Hand Yang Ming Large Intestine

Foot Jue Yin Liver

"That was impressive, Sun. You are an excellent student. Now we think about the images. What images can you think of for the ankle?"

"Well, the ankle is on the leg, and the leg can image to the other leg or the arm. If I use the leg to image the leg I would use the other ankle and perhaps the hip. The hip because it is the reversed image of the leg. On the arm, I would think about the wrist and the shoulder."

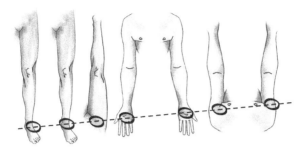

left leg   left leg   right leg right arm left arm   left arm   right arm

"Perfect. Now you can palpate the interacting channels on the ankles, hips, wrists, and shoulders. And remember that some systems need to be on the opposite side."

"Yes, Systems 1, 2, and 4 are on the opposite side. I remember that. But this seems like a lot of palpating. Is there not a more direct way?"

"Well, there is. A second approach is to do all the logic as we said before, look at all the possible channel interactions and images, but then think about which have the most similar anatomical structures. You start by palpating those. Where would that be for you in this case?"

"I would think the other ankle is very similar and perhaps also the wrists. So that is where I would look."

"Very good. The ankles are of course very similar; however, the only system that could use the other ankle is System 1 Interior/Exterior. And here we would be on the Foot Shao Yang Gall Bladder at the ankle and the problem is on the Foot Jue Yin Liver channel. Because one is on the Yin side and the other on the Yang side, the anatomical similarity is less. With the wrists it is better. And as the other five channels that interact with the Foot Jue Yin Liver are all arm channels, they pass through the wrist. So, in this case you could palpate the interacting channels at the wrist and use the most sensitive. We would just need to remember that Systems

2 and 4 are on the opposite side. So, we could palpate the channels on the opposite side to make it easier."

"OK, that makes sense. If I were to think in steps it would be like this:

Step 1: Identify the problem.

Step 2: Identify the channel that the problem is on.

Step 3: Look at the six systems and which channels interact with the channel that has the problem.

Step 4: Take the area where the problem is and image it onto the interacting channels.

Step 5: Figure out which images have the most anatomical similarities and start palpating there.

Step 6: Palpate the channels and images to find the most sensitive points and use those."

"Excellent. That is the general way to approach it. Now there is another way to navigate the whole system, which comes from years of experience using these ideas. To do this we will make a bunch of statements about the systems and how they interact, and from these statements we will see patterns that emerge."

"OK. So, this is the advanced stuff! Let's have it."

"Haha! Well, let's say experienced instead of advanced.

- There are six Yin channels.

- There are six Yang channels.

- There are six foot channels.

- There are six hand channels.

- There are six channel interaction systems:
  - three systems based on time
  - two systems based on tine
  - one system based on sunlight.
- Systems 1, 2, and 4 all only have one basic polarity so must be used contra-laterally.
- Systems 3, 5, and 6 all have both basic polarities so can be used either side.
- System 1 is the only system to stay on the same limb.

"And now let's add some more complexity:

- Systems 2 and 4 are the same for all the Yang channels.
- Systems 5 and 6 are the same for the Yin channels of the hand and the Yang channels of the foot.

"Based on this information we can say the following.

"As the Yin channels of the foot do not have any systems that repeat, they have six possible interactions:

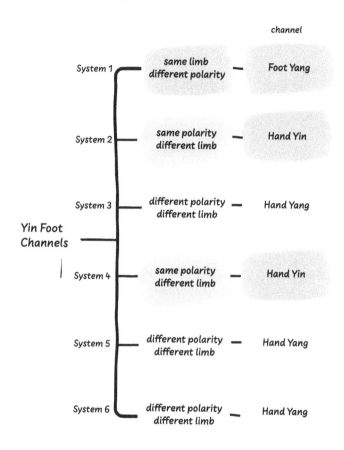

"As the Yin channels of the hand have one repeating pair of interactions, they have five possible interactions:

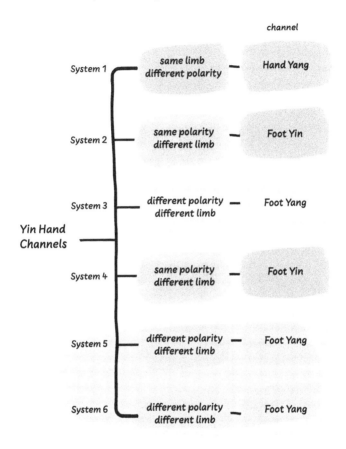

"As the Yang channels of the hand have one repeating pair of interactions, they have five possible interactions:

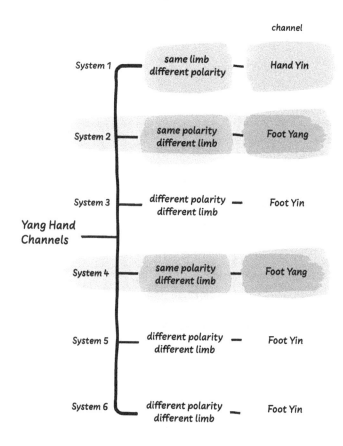

channel

System 1 — **same limb different polarity** — **Hand Yin**

System 2 — **same polarity different limb** — **Foot Yang**

System 3 — **different polarity different limb** — Foot Yin

Yang Hand Channels

System 4 — **same polarity different limb** — **Foot Yang**

System 5 — **different polarity different limb** — Foot Yin

System 6 — **different polarity different limb** — Foot Yin

"As the Yang channels of the leg have two repeating systems, they have four possible interactions:

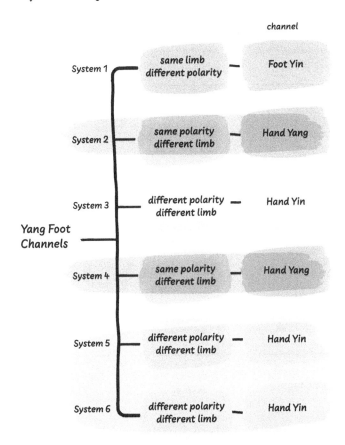

channel

System 1	same limb different polarity	Foot Yin
System 2	same polarity different limb	Hand Yang
System 3	different polarity different limb	Hand Yin
System 4	same polarity different limb	Hand Yang
System 5	different polarity different limb	Hand Yin
System 6	different polarity different limb	Hand Yin

Yang Foot Channels

"So, we can say that the arms have ten interactions: five on the Yin channels and five on the Yang channels.

"The legs have ten interactions also, but distributed differently: six on the Yin channels and four on the Yang channels."

Sun was listening and looking. "OK, so far so good."

"Great. Now if we take all this together, we will see that

any foot Yin channel will interact with all the Yang channels of the foot and any Yang channel of the hand will interact with all the Yin channels of the foot.

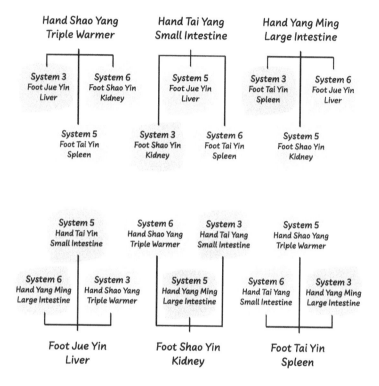

"So, if we have a problem on two or more Yin channels, we can take any Yang channel of the arm, and vice versa.

"Also, any two Yin channels when put together will treat all the Yin channels of the arm."

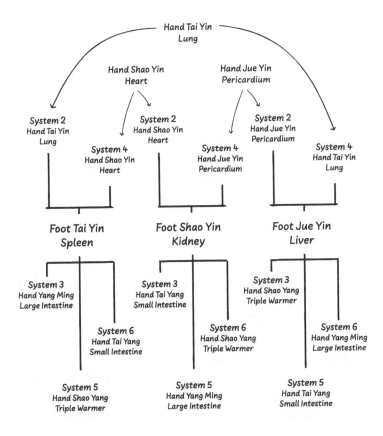

Sun was impressed. "So, if I have a problem in the arm, I can always just take two Yin channels of the foot and I know I will treat the problem."

"That is correct, Sun. This is why the Yin channels on the foot are so useful. Now, if the problem is only on one channel in the arm, it is better to go through all the different systems to find the best point, like we did before, as this gives the most options and the most similar anatomical structure. But when there is more than one channel involved in the problem, then yes, taking any two Yin channels of the foot is a shortcut.

"And we can also add that any two Yin channels of the foot together will interact with all the channels of the hand and four channels of the foot."

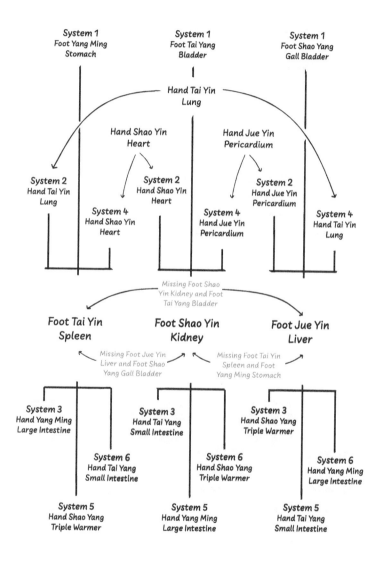

"OK, this makes it easier. I will have to study these connections more."

"That is normal, Sun. It is when you start using the systems that you start to integrate all this information. This comes from practice. That is why we often do not teach this in the beginner course because it would be too confusing. We are adding it here, with you, so you can integrate it slowly. There is one more statement to add.

"Any three channels of the same limb and same polarity will treat all the other channels of the body. You can see this if you add all the previous images together.

"So, a summary of the shortcuts would be the following:

- All the Yin channels of the foot interact with all three Yang channels of the hand.

- All the Yang channels of the hand interact with all three Yin channels of the foot.

- Any two Yin channels of the foot interact with all the channels of the hand.

- Any two Yin channels of the hand interact with all the channels of the foot.

- Any two channels of the same polarity (Yin/Yang) and the same limb in addition to any channel that is based on space (Systems 1, 2, and 3) of the omitted channel on the limb will interact with all the channels of the body.

- All three channels of the same polarity (Yin/Yang) and the same limb will interact with all the channels of the body."

"Brilliant, I think I need some time to digest all of this."

Grandfather Terra filled the teacups and said, "That is very wise of you, Sun."

CHAPTER 21

A Guiding Light

The Guiding Needle Technique

The penultimate day of Sun's stay had arrived. They knew that tomorrow they would be going home. They were not as sad as they would have been because they knew that their grandparents were going to be in their hometown more often. Sun got up and went downstairs for the morning Qi Gong exercises. Sun really enjoyed doing these and could feel themselves getting stronger. When they had finished with the routine, Grandmother Terra brought out three planks of wood. She held one up between her hands and Grandfather Terra punched right through it. Sun was amazed. They never imagined their grandfather having so much strength. And then they got even more amazed when Grandfather Terra held up the wooden plank and Grandmother Terra punched right through it. Sun realized that their grandparents were superheroes.

Then Grandmother Terra picked up the last plank and held it up for Sun. "Sun, now it is your turn."

"What? Are you serious? I can't punch through that."

Grandfather Terra was chuckling. "I know it seems impossible Sun, but we are going to share a trick with you. The key to it is where you aim. If you aim for the plank, it will be impossible. But if you aim 15cm behind the plank you will come at the plank with all your force and will succeed. Now get into the punching stance we showed you from the Qi Gong. Center yourself and feel the Qi in your lower abdomen. When you are ready, you punch aiming behind the plank and exhale at the same time."

Sun thought they were crazy. There was no way they would be able to punch through the wood. But Sun had learned to trust their grandparents. They centered themselves and breathed deeply. They took their concentration down into their abdomen and felt the warmth come from there. They then imagined punching 15cm further than the wood that Grandmother Terra was holding in front of them. With a large exhale they punched forward with all their might. Crack! They had done it! Sun was so pleased. Both grandparents were smiling and clapping. Sun had become a superhero as well.

They spent the rest of the day enjoying their normal activities: gardening, going for a walk, and finally having tea. When they were comfortably sitting on the porch and drinking the warm liquid, Sun started a conversation.

"I think I have understood how the channels interact and how the distal points can have actions that are far away from where they are, but there is one thing that I was thinking about. For example, the case of yesterday with the ankle problem on the Foot Jue Yin Liver channel. We saw that the Hand Yang Ming Large Intestine at the wrist would be a good treatment. Well, that point there also interacts with a bunch of other channels as well, and a bunch of other images. How does it know to treat the Foot Jue Yin Liver at the ankle?"

Grandmother Terra answered, "An interesting question, and an apt one too. Yes, each point can have many effects on the body. They can interact with anywhere from four to six other channels and their own channel as well. So, the first thing we can say is that the body is very intelligent, and when there is a problem on the Foot Jue Yin Liver and we place a needle on the Hand Yang Ming Large Intestine channel, it knows how to use that information. There is also a way we can help it. This is called the Guiding Needle Technique."

"What is that?"

Grandmother Terra responded, "It is a way to guide the Qi to the problem area. We do this by adding a needle to guide the Qi to where we want it to interact. There are some guidelines on how to do this:

- We place the guiding needle point on the affected channel.

- We place the guiding needle more distal than the affected area.

- We have two options on how to choose which needle:

  - We can use what is called the Ying-Spring point or the Shu-Stream point.

  - We can choose an image on the affected channel that is more distal than the problem.

"So, let's look at a new problem and go through all the steps and add the guiding needle to see how it works.

"A person has what is called tennis elbow. This is a pain at the elbow on the Hand Yang Ming Large Intestine channel. The pain is normally on the bone. Let's say it is on the right hand."

Sun nodded. "OK. So, you already did the first step for me. The diagnosis is Hand Yang Ming Large Intestine at the right elbow. The Hand Yang Ming Large Intestine is a Yang channel of the hand, so it has five interactions. System 2 Full Channels and System 4 Biorhythm Neighbors are the same for all the Yang channels.

"The channels that interact with the Hand Yang Ming Large Intestine are:

System 1: Hand Tai Yin Lung

System 2: Foot Yang Ming Stomach

System 3: Foot Tai Yin Spleen

System 4: Foot Yang Ming Stomach (same as System 2)

System 5: Foot Shao Yin Liver

System 6: Foot Jue Yin Liver.

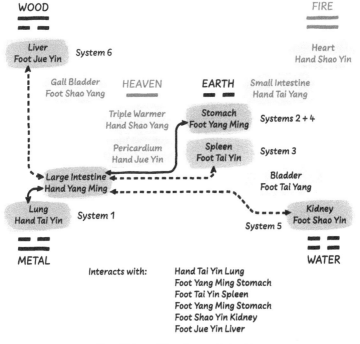

Hand Yang Ming Large Intestine

"OK, now for the images. The elbow is the middle joint on the arm and can image onto the other arm and the leg. The middle joint of the other arm is also the elbow and of the leg is the knee."

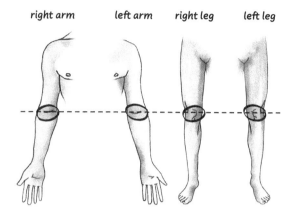

Grandfather Terra was pleased. "Very good. And now let's put the images with the channels."

"OK, let me think.

System 1: Hand Tai Yin Lung—opposite elbow

System 2: Foot Yang Ming Stomach—opposite knee

System 3: Foot Tai Yin Spleen—either knee

System 4: Foot Yang Ming Stomach (same as System 2)—opposite knee

System 5: Foot Shao Yin Liver—either knee

System 6: Foot Jue Yin Liver—either knee.

"I said for the Hand Tai Yin Lung and the Foot Yang Ming Stomach it had to be on the opposite side because Systems 1, 2, and 4 are all opposite side systems."

"Excellent. So now we think about which of these possibilities has the most similar anatomical structure to the Hand Yang Ming Large Intestine at the elbow. A good way to do this is to first put your finger at the place where the problem is and feel what is there. Is there bone, tendons, muscle, and so on? What do you feel at the elbow where the problem is?"

"I feel that there is a bone and some muscle."

"And now, if you feel for the interacting channels at the knee and elbow, which feels the most similar?"

Sun touched all their joints and compared them. "I would say that the Foot Jue Yin Liver is the most similar. It is also next to a bone and has a tendon near it too."

"Very good. I agree with you. Now let's add the guiding needle to the treatment to help the body to use the needle at the knee on the Foot Jue Yin Liver channel to treat the elbow and the Hand Yang Ming channel. Do you remember how to do this?"

"Honestly, not really. Could you walk me through it?"

"Of course. The first step is to add the needle to the affected channel and on the same side. So, we will look for a point on the right Hand Yang Ming Large Intestine channel. Now we will look for a point that is more distal than the problem. So, we will look on the right Hand Yang Ming Large Intestine channel more distal than the elbow."

Sun asked, "Why does the guiding needle have to be more distal? Would it not call the Qi to the area better if it were where the problem is?"

"That is a question we are asked a lot. Let's think about this morning when we broke the wooden planks. Did we aim for the plank or behind the plank?"

"We aimed behind the plank, so we would have our full force when we struck the plank."

"It is the same thing here. We are guiding the Qi to move through the problem and continue after it. This pulls the Qi all the way through the problem and helps the general circulation.

"So, let's move to where more distally we will place the guiding needle.

"We have two choices: either the Ying-Spring or Shu-Stream point, or an image of the elbow that is further away."

"Well, the Ying-Spring and Shu-Stream points are set points, I imagine. And as for an image, I thought that only the elbow imaged the elbow in the arm."

"You are correct for the Ying-Spring and Shu-Stream points. The Ying-Spring point is Erijian LI 2 and the Shu-Stream point is Sanjian LI 3. These are on both sides of the metacarpal-phalangeal joint on the index finger.

"For an image we can also use what we call the small Taiji images. Do you remember using a bone for the whole arm? Here we can use the metacarpal bone of the hand to image the whole arm."

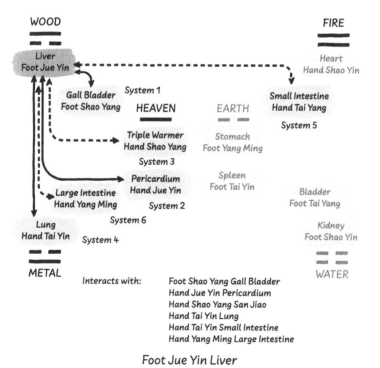

Foot Jue Yin Liver

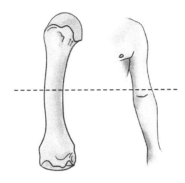

Sun looked at this image. "I had forgotten about this idea. OK. So, this will be in the middle of the bone because that is what images the elbow. Is there an acupuncture point here?"

"It is normal to forget about this image. It is a more advanced image, and it becomes very useful when using the guiding needle. There is an acupuncture point here. It is Hegu LI 4 and it is one of the most used points in acupuncture. Even if there was no acupuncture point here, you could still use it as it is the image.

"So, let's sum up the treatment:

Diagnosis: Hand Yang Ming Large Intestine on the right side.

Interacting Channels with their images:

System 1: Hand Tai Yin Lung—opposite elbow

System 2: Foot Yang Ming Stomach—opposite knee

System 3: Foot Tai Yin Spleen—either knee

System 4: Foot Yang Ming Stomach (same as System 2)—opposite knee

System 5: Foot Shao Yin Liver—either knee

System 6: Foot Jue Yin Liver—either knee.

Best choice: System 6: Foot Jue Yin Liver—either knee.

Guiding needle: On the right side: Erijian LI 2, Sanjian LI 3, or Hegu LI 4.

"That is it."

Sun understood. "OK, that seems simple enough. For the guiding needle, I see the idea of the image, but I do not understand why those Ying-Spring and Shu-Stream points are used."

"Well, Sun, that is a good question. These points are part of what we call the five transporting points. Every channel has these points and they describe the density of the Qi flowing in that area of the channel. They use the image of a water way. The most distal point is called a Jing-Well point, then moving toward the body they are the Ying-Spring point, Shu-Stream point, Jing-River point, and He-Sea point. So, let's imagine that you hurt yourself and wanted to wash in the water. Which of these is the easiest to wash away your pain?"

"I guess it would be the spring and the river points. The well would be too deep to access, the river too dangerous, and the sea too salty. The spring and the stream are both gentle enough to wash in and the water is very fresh too."

"Excellent. So that is the idea."

Grandfather Terra asked, "More tea anyone?"

CHAPTER 22

WHEN FAMILY MATTERS

Using Channel Interactions, Imaging, and the Family of Points Together

Once the tea had been poured Sun jumped right back in. "I have another question. We have talked about using palpation and imaging to choose the best treatment. I remember that at the beginning of the summer you also mentioned the family of points. You said that with them combined with the channel interactions and the imaging we could understand most point indications. Can we also use the family of points to help choose the best treatment?"

Grandfather Terra answered, "Yes, Sun, we can. It is good that you remembered that point, as that is where we started on this adventure. How about this, we first look at the families of points, try to understand them, and then see how they fit in. Do you remember the different types of points we talked about?"

"To be honest, not really. They are all vague in my mind."

"OK, let's see them again.

- Five Element points

- On each main channel, there will be a point that is associated with one of the five elements. We studied these elements last summer. They are fire, earth, metal, water, and wood. These points will bring the quality of their associated element to the channel that they are placed on. So, for example, on the Foot Shao Yan Kidney channel there will be one point of each element. We know the Kidney is associated with the water element. This means that if we use the point associated with metal on the water element it will bring the metal energy into water and the Kidneys. This is the basis of what is called five element acupuncture.

- In addition to each of these points having an element associated with them, their position going from most distal to most proximal also has a name and a use. We saw them when we looked at the guiding needle point. They represent a water way going from a well, to a spring, to a stream, to a river, and finally to the sea. The more distal the point, the newer information the point can have on the body. The more proximal, the more the point reinforces the function of the channel or organ.

- Yuan or Source points
  - This group of points is often grouped with the Five Element points and together they are given the name Shu or transporting points. Each channel has one of these points. On the Yin channels they are the same as the point that is associated with the earth point, and on the Yang channels they are normally placed between the wood and the fire points. These points are used to remind the channel

and the associated organ of their original function. There is a type of Qi called Yuan or Source Qi that is strong in these points.

- Luo or Connecting points

  - In each element there is a pairing of a Yin and Yang organ and channel, as well as many other associations. These associations include the sense organs in the face. This group of points are the communicators between the Yin-Yang pairs in the element and the sense organs in the head. For example, the metal element has the Hand Tai Yin channel, which is associated with the Lung, and the Hand Yang Ming channel, which is associated with the Large Intestine. These two channels together are also associated with the nose on the face. The connecting point on the Yin channel will connect with the Yang channel at the Source point. The connecting point of the Yang channel will connect with the face.

- Xi or Cleft points

  - These points are also known as emergency points. Each channel has one of these points and it helps the channel when it is in an emergency. That means when the channel really needs help.

"These are the family of points we saw earlier."

"Yes, I remember them now."

"Good. So, we can use these points to help us decide. Let's give an example. A person has a burning feeling at the base of their left toe on the inner part. We would say that it is Foot Tai Yin Spleen that is affected. How would you go through the rest of the treatment?"

"Well, I would look at which channels interact with the Foot Tai Yin Spleen.

System 1: Foot Yang Ming Stomach

System 2: Hand Tai Yin Lung

System 3: Hand Yang Ming Large Intestine

System 4: Hand Shao Yin Heart

System 5: Hand Shao Yang Triple Warmer

System 6: Hand Tai Yang Small Intestine.

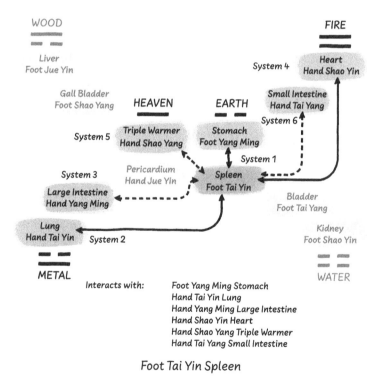

Interacts with: Foot Yang Ming Stomach
Hand Tai Yin Lung
Hand Yang Ming Large Intestine
Hand Shao Yin Heart
Hand Shao Yang Triple Warmer
Hand Tai Yang Small Intestine

Foot Tai Yin Spleen

"Next, I would look at the images. The foot can be the hand or the other foot.

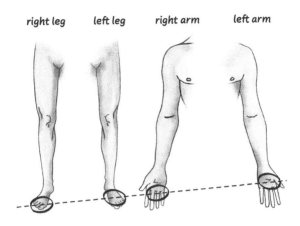

right leg   **left leg**   **right arm**   **left arm**

"So, I would look at the following:

System 1: Foot Yang Ming Stomach—opposite foot

System 2: Hand Tai Yin Lung—opposite hand

System 3: Hand Yang Ming Large Intestine—either hand

System 4: Hand Shao Yin Heart—opposite hand

System 5: Hand Shao Yang Triple Warmer—either hand

System 6: Hand Tai Yang Small Intestine—either hand."

Grandmother Terra spoke, "That is perfect, Sun. Now we can look for which has the most similar anatomical structure. And we would probably say that it is the thumb on the hand, which would be either the Foot Tai Yin Lung or the Hand Yang Ming Large Intestine. So, to help us decide more, we would look at if any of the family of points are in this area and if they make sense to treat the problem. We would find that on the base of the thumb on the Hand Tai Yin Lung there is the point LU 10 Yuji. This point is the Ying-Spring and the fire point on the Hand Tai Yin Lung channel. Now the problem the patient has is a burning sensation. So, this burning sensation and a fire point go well together. So, we would choose this point."

Sun was nodding. "I see now. If I take the qualities of the family of points and if I find that the image is close to these points, then I can take that into account. I guess it only works when the image matches up?"

"Exactly. We add the family of points to our decision-making process only after we have seen the images and the channel interactions. They can help us decide between two or three possibilities."

"And what about a guiding needle in this case?"

"Well, as the problem is at the toe, it is difficult to add a point that is more distal, meaning further away from the body. So, in some cases, especially when it is on the hands or feet, we do not add the guiding needle. It does not always need to be used."

CHAPTER 23

WHEN IT GETS COMPLICATED

Case Studies Involving More Than One Affected Channel

Sun was thinking about the families of points and how they could add the information into the treatment when Grandfather Terra spoke. "Let's take a look at some more difficult cases and see what we can do. Here is a person who has pain in the elbow, thigh, and a headache. If you look at the image here, you can see where the pain is.

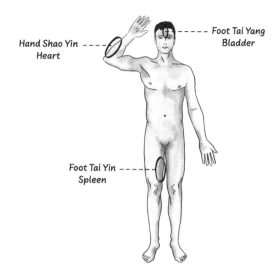

"Here we have three different problems on three different channels. How do you think you would treat this?"

Sun looked at the image. "This is more complicated. I am not sure how to go about it. If it were only one problem, or one channel, then I could figure it out, but here I am not sure."

"Well, the steps are always the same, no matter how complicated the problem is.

Step 1: Identify the affected channel or channels.

Step 2: See which channels interact with the affected channel or channels.

Step 3: Apply the images and mirroring.

"Step 1 we did. The affected channels are:

Foot Tai Yin Spleen

Foot Tai Yang Bladder

Hand Shao Yin Heart.

"Step 2 is the interacting channels."

"OK, so I will do each one on its own then I guess:

Foot Tai Yin Spleen

System 1: Foot Yang Ming Stomach—opposite side

System 2: Hand Tai Yin Lung—opposite side

System 3: Hand Yang Ming Large Intestine—either side

System 4: Hand Shao Yin Heart—opposite side

System 5: Hand Shao Yang Triple Warmer—either side

System 6: Hand Tai Yang Small Intestine—either side.

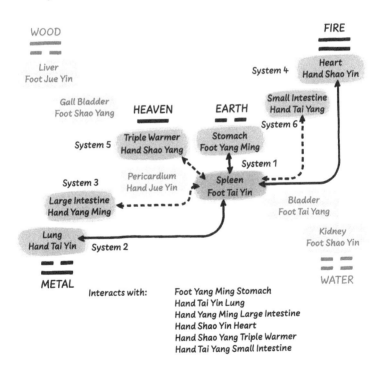

Foot Tai Yang Bladder

System 1: Foot Shao Yin Kidney—opposite side

System 2: Hand Tai Yang Small Intestine—opposite side

System 3: Hand Shao Yin Heart—either side

System 4: Hand Tai Yang Small Intestine—opposite side (Systems 2 and 4 are the same for Yang channels)

System 5: Hand Tai Yin Lung—either side

System 6: Hand Tai Yin Lung—either side (Systems 5 and 6 are the same for Yang foot and Yin hand channels).

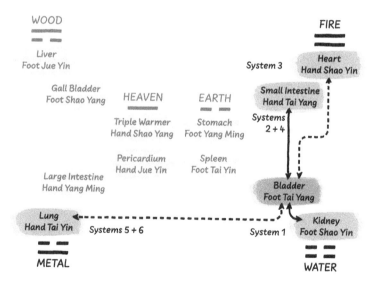

Hand Shao Yin Heart

System 1: Hand Tai Yang Small Intestine—opposite side

System 2: Foot Shao Yin Kidney—opposite side

System 3: Foot Tai Yang Bladder—either side

System 4: Foot Tai Yin Spleen—opposite side

System 5: Foot Shao Yang Gall Bladder—either side

System 6: Foot Shao Yang Gall Bladder—either side (Systems 5 and 6 are the same for Yang foot and Yin hand channels).

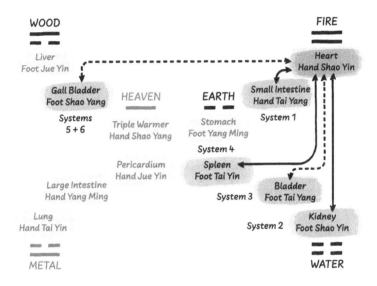

"OK, and now that I have all these channel interactions?"

"Well now, we see if there are any channels that interact with all three affected channels. Can you find any?"

Sun looked at all three charts for a moment and then said, "I found one. The Hand Tai Yang Small Intestine. It interacts with all three channels.

"Hand Tai Yang Small Intestine interacts with:

Foot Tai Yin Spleen: System 6 Exposure to Sunlight— either side

Foot Tai Yang Bladder: System 2 Full Channels—opposite side

Hand Shao Yin Heart: System 1 Interior/Exterior—opposite side.

"So, the channel is the Hand Tai Yang Small Intestine."

"Very good, Sun. You have found one channel that interacts with all three affected channels. Now let's image the problems onto the Hand Tai Yang Small Intestine."

"OK. Let me see. I will do each one separately. The problem on the Foot Tai Yin Spleen was on the thigh. This can be either above or below the elbow on the Hand Tai Yang Small Intestine.

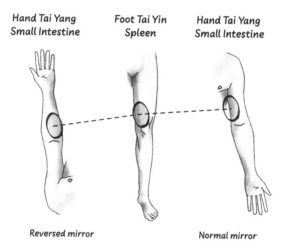

Hand Tai Yang   Foot Tai Yin   Hand Tai Yang
Small Intestine   Spleen   Small Intestine

Reversed mirror   Normal mirror

"The problem on the Foot Tai Yang Bladder was above the eye on the head. This can be either above or below the elbow on the Hand Tai Yang Small Intestine, as the level is the same as the elbow.

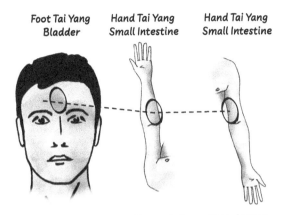

Foot Tai Yang Bladder Hand Tai Yang Small Intestine Hand Tai Yang Small Intestine

Reversed mirror   Normal mirror

"And finally, the problem on the Hand Shao Yin Heart was on the elbow. So we use the elbow on the Hand Tai Yang Small Intestine.

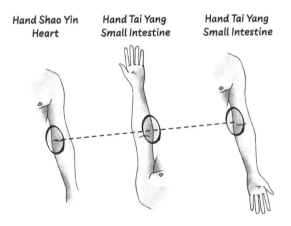

Hand Shao Yin Heart Hand Tai Yang Small Intestine Hand Tai Yang Small Intestine

Reversed mirror   Normal mirror

"That is all."

"That is very good, Sun. So, let's put it all together. How would you do that?"

"Well, I would take the Hand Tai Yang Small Intestine to treat all three problem channels. I would put needles from the elbow to the middle of the forearm. The needles at the elbow would treat the elbow problem on the Hand Shao Yin Heart channel, and the needles from the elbow to the middle of the forearm would treat the problems on the Foot Tai Yin Spleen and the Foot Tai Yang Bladder channels."

"Which side would you put the needles on?"

"As all the problems were on the right side of the body, I would use the left side for the Hand Tai Yang Small Intestine because it interacts with Hand Shao Yin Heart with System 1 Interior/Exterior and Foot Tai Yang Bladder with System 2 Full Channels. Both of these interactions must be opposite side as they are either on the same limb or Yin-Yang polarity as the Hand Tai Yang Small Intestine channel."

"Perfect, Sun. You just took a difficult problem with three different channels and found a simple treatment with only using one channel. Very well done. Should we do another one?"

"Of course we should. Do you expect me to say no?"

"Haha! OK. This time we will make it even more complicated. But we will still follow the same logic.

"A patient comes in with Bell's Palsy on the left side of the face. This means that the left side of the face has become paralyzed. Walk us through the logic."

"Wow, that sounds serious. OK, I need to ask, which channels are touched by the problem?"

"It sounds serious, and it does happen quite often. Your question is the perfect one. All the channels of the head except for the Foot Tai Yang Bladder channel are affected."

"So, all the channels in the head are Yang, so that means the channels that are touched are the:

Hand Tai Yang Small Intestine

Hand Yang Ming Large Intestine

Hand Shao Yang Triple Warmer

Foot Yang Ming Stomach

Foot Shao Yang Gall Bladder.

"I have a feeling this would be a good time to use the short-cuts we talked about. It would take a lot of time to do it channel by channel."

"Yes, Sun. This is a good case to use the shortcuts on. First, look at the problem channels and see what you can say about them."

"Well, they are all Yang channels. They are all three in the hand and only two in the foot."

"Very good. So, what did we say about the hand Yang channels?"

"We said that every hand Yang channel interacts with all the foot Yin channels."

"Good. Let's use the foot Yin channels. We still have the two foot Yang channels to work with."

"Well, any two Yin channels of the hand will interact with all the Yang channels of the foot. And each Yin channel of the hand interacts with two different Yang channels of the foot."

"Yes, that is true. So, we could find the Yin channel of the hand that interacts with both the Foot Shao Yang Gall Bladder and the Foot Yang Ming Stomach. Which channel is that?"

"I cannot think about it that quickly. Give me a second while I look at the charts."

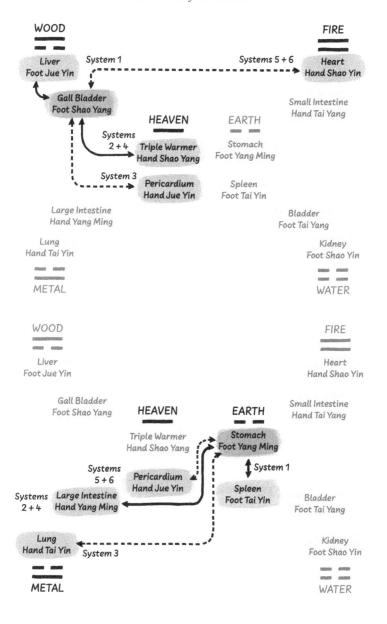

Sun looked and said, "The Hand Jue Yin Pericardium interacts with both."

"Very good, Sun. So, we can use any of the foot Yin channels with the Hand Jue Yin Pericardium and we will interact with all five affected channels. Now there is another option as well. Since all three Yin of the legs interact with all the Yang of the arms, we need to use at least one Yin foot channel. Each foot channel also has one interaction with a Yang foot channel. So, if we choose two Yin foot channels, we will interact with all the Yang of the hand and two Yang of the foot. Look at the images again for the Foot Shao Yang Gall Bladder and the Foot Yang Ming Stomach. Which Yin foot channels do they interact with?"

Sun looked. "That is easier, as it is System 1 Interior/Exterior and I know that system the best. Foot Shao Yang Gall Bladder interacts with Foot Jue Yin Liver, and the Foot Yang Ming Stomach interacts with Foot Tai Yin Spleen."

"Very good. So now we have two possibilities for the interacting channels. We can choose either one Yin channel of the foot and the Hand Jue Yin Pericardium or the Foot Tai Yin Spleen and the Foot Jue Yin Liver. Both of these will work."

"Could I choose both together? I mean, could I use all three channels: Foot Jue Yin Liver, Foot Tai Yin Spleen, and Hand Jue Yin Pericardium?"

"Yes, you can. In fact, that is often the best approach. This way you are interacting with each affected channel at least twice. And now what about the imaging? Where would you put the needles on the three channels?"

"The problem is in the face, so I will use the image of the head to the limbs. So, I would need to use the whole limb to image the whole head."

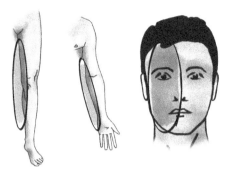

"This is a possibility, and we can do it. However, we can reduce the number of points by combining the normal and the reversed images.

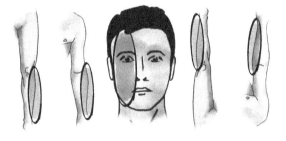

"Here we have the forearms and the lower leg imaging from the eyes to the chin on the normal image. When we reverse the image, the forearm and the lower leg are now imaging the eyes to the top of the head. So, we can reduce by only using half the limb to treat the whole head."

Sun nodded. "OK, so our treatment will be needles from the wrist to the elbow on the Hand Jue Yin Liver channel, and needles from the ankle to the knee on the Foot Jue Yin Liver and Foot Tai Yin Spleen channels. All would be on the right side as the problem is on the left and some of the interactions must be opposite side. Would we add a guiding needle?"

"Yes. Here we could add points on the hands and the feet on the same side as the problem. The hands and the feet are images of the head. So, for the following, this is what we would probably use:

> Hand Yang Ming Large Intestine—LI 4 Hegu. This is the Yuan source point and the command point of the face.
>
> Hand Tai Yang Small Intestine—SI 3 Houxi. This is the Shu-Stream point and the opening point of the Du Mai.
>
> Hand Shao Yang Triple Warmer—TW 3 Zhong Zhu. This is the Shu-Stream point.
>
> Foot Yang Ming Stomach—ST 43 Xian Gu. This is the Shu-Stream point.
>
> Foot Shao Yang Gall Bladder—GB 41 Zu Lin Qi. This is the Shu-Stream point.

"All the Shu-Stream points on the Yang channels are wood points. In traditional Chinese medicine, facial paralysis is seen as a wind problem and the element wood is associated with treating wind."

"Wow, that all fits together. It seems complicated and easy at the same time. I mean, if I didn't have the logic to understand, it would seem way too difficult, but I feel as if I can grasp it and see how it works, even if I can't do it as fast as you guys can."

Grandfather Terra was smiling. "That's normal, Sun. We have spent our lives using and understanding this. It is almost second nature to us. You will need to practice and use it for it to become more alive. That is why we have created this for you."

Grandmother Terra gave Sun a package. It was wrapped in beautiful red rice paper and had "For Sun" written in big letters.

"Thank you very much," Sun said while they carefully opened the parcel. It was a handmade book, just like last time. This time it said *The Unified Acupuncture Theory: Quick Reference Book, by Grandparents Terra.* It had a beautiful image of what looked like a circle and the Yin-Yang lines all at the same time.

Sun looked up with a big smile and gave both grandparents a big hug. "Thank you both very much. I love it."

CHAPTER 24

SUN GOES HOME

Conclusion

Dinner was a simple affair. They prepared some of Sun's favorite foods and made sure there was leftovers for sandwiches for the train ride the next day. They talked lightly about the summer and how they were happy to spend time in each other's company. There was not the heaviness that they felt the previous summer, as they knew they would be seeing each other more often now that the grandparents were going to start teaching again at the university.

After the meal had been cleared away and the tidying up done, they went to sit on the porch one last time as it was a perfect evening for porch sitting.

Sun looked up at the sky and was deep in thoughts when Grandmother Terra started to speak. "So tomorrow you will be going home, Sun. How do you feel about going back to your school and your life there?"

Sun came out of their daze and took a second to gather their thoughts. "I am not quite sure how I feel. I have had a very good summer here with you two. I have learned a lot about acupuncture and also about myself. I feel as if I am stronger than I was at the beginning of the summer. And I also know that you two will be in town more often, so I will get to see my two favorite teachers more regularly."

Grandfather Terra said, "That is all true, Sun. You have learned a lot about acupuncture and yourself. And you will see us more. And these are all mental statements about what you think." Grandmother Terra asked, "How do you feel?"

Sun avoided looking at Grandmother Terra as they took in her words. "How do I feel? There are many feelings happening at the same time. I am happy that I was here for the summer. I am sad that I am leaving and will miss you. I am anxious about going back to school and a little bit scared of life back home, and I am excited to think about seeing you in town."

Grandmother Terra got up and walked over to Sun and asked them to stand up. Sun got up, and before they could know what was happening, Grandmother Terra had Sun in a big hug. She held Sun there until she felt Sun's body relax and finally accept being hugged. Then she looked Sun in the eyes and said, "You are really an exceptional person, Sun. We are so proud to be your grandparents. We love you, Sun."

All three of them went to bed with happy tears for the summer they had shared. The next day they all got up, did their Qi Gong together, had breakfast, and got ready to go to the train station. No one felt like talking, so they all went about in comfortable silence.

Waiting on the platform, they all hugged but remained silent. As the train pulled up and Sun got on, Sun looked back at both grandparents, and in a loud voice said, "Thank you for a wonderful summer. I love you both. See you very soon for more lessons."

Both grandparents were smiling and looking forward to teaching Sun everything they knew.

THE UNIFIED ACUPUNCTURE THEORY

Quick Reference Book

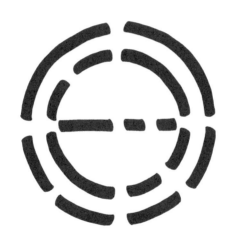

by
Grandparents Terra

THE SYSTEMS

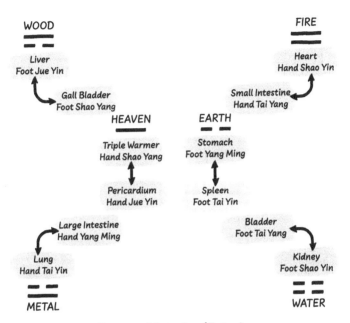

System 1 Interior/Exterior

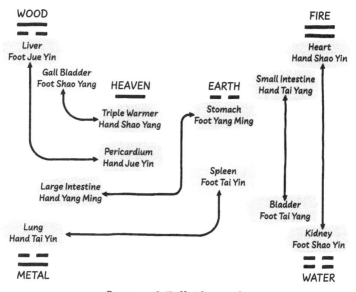

System 2 Full Channels

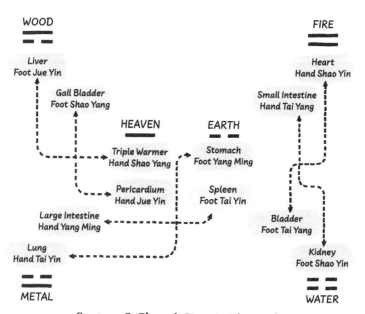

System 3 Closed Circuit Channels

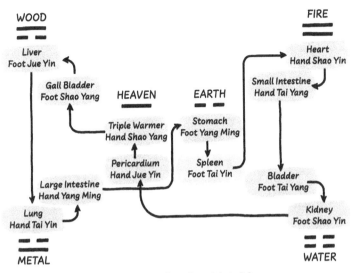

System 4 Biorhythm Neighbors

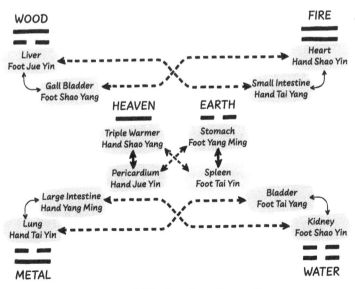

System 5 Biorhythm Opposites

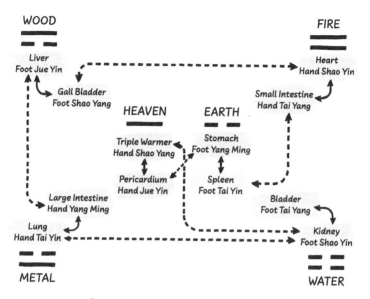

System 6 Exposure to Sunlight

A REFERENCE FOR INTERACTIONS OF EACH CHANNEL

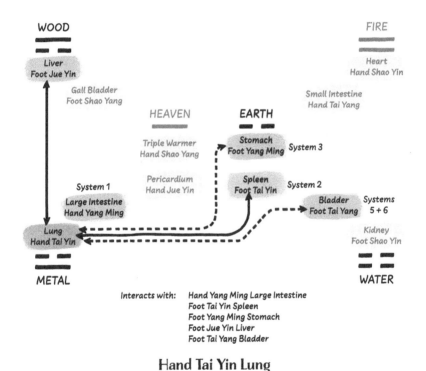

WOOD

Liver
Foot Jue Yin

Gall Bladder
Foot Shao Yang

HEAVEN

Triple Warmer
Hand Shao Yang

Pericardium
Hand Jue Yin

System 1

Large Intestine
Hand Yang Ming

Lung
Hand Tai Yin

METAL

EARTH

Stomach
Foot Yang Ming   System 3

Spleen
Foot Tai Yin   System 2

Bladder   Systems
Foot Tai Yang   5 + 6

FIRE

Heart
Hand Shao Yin

Small Intestine
Hand Tai Yang

Kidney
Foot Shao Yin

WATER

Interacts with: Hand Yang Ming Large Intestine
Foot Tai Yin Spleen
Foot Yang Ming Stomach
Foot Jue Yin Liver
Foot Tai Yang Bladder

Hand Tai Yin Lung

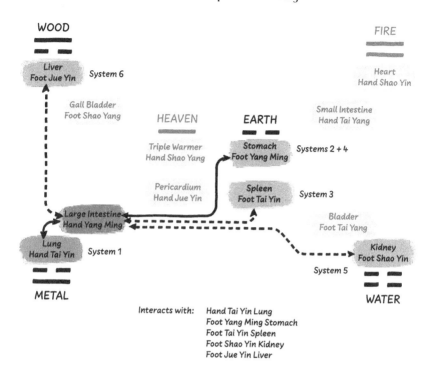

Hand Yang Ming Large Intestine

A Reference for Interactions of Each Channel

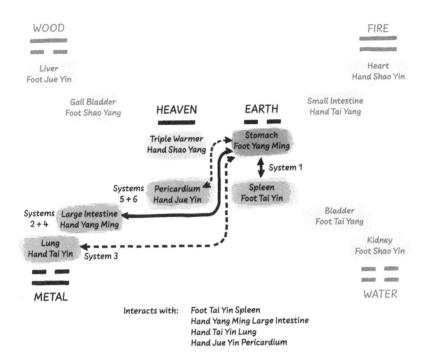

WOOD

Liver
Foot Jue Yin

FIRE

Heart
Hand Shao Yin

Gall Bladder
Foot Shao Yang

HEAVEN

EARTH

Small Intestine
Hand Tai Yang

Triple Warmer
Hand Shao Yang

Stomach
Foot Yang Ming

System 1

Systems
5 + 6

Pericardium
Hand Jue Yin

Spleen
Foot Tai Yin

Bladder
Foot Tai Yang

Systems
2 + 4

Large Intestine
Hand Yang Ming

Kidney
Foot Shao Yin

Lung
Hand Tai Yin   System 3

METAL

WATER

Interacts with: Foot Tai Yin Spleen
Hand Yang Ming Large Intestine
Hand Tai Yin Lung
Hand Jue Yin Pericardium

Foot Yang Ming Stomach

The Unified Acupuncture Theory

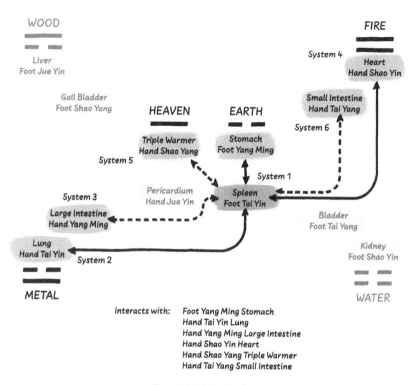

WOOD

Liver
Foot Jue Yin

Gall Bladder
Foot Shao Yang

HEAVEN

EARTH

FIRE

System 4

Heart
Hand Shao Yin

Small Intestine
Hand Tai Yang

System 6

Triple Warmer
Hand Shao Yang

Stomach
Foot Yang Ming

System 5

System 1

System 3

Pericardium
Hand Jue Yin

Spleen
Foot Tai Yin

Large Intestine
Hand Yang Ming

Bladder
Foot Tai Yang

Lung
Hand Tai Yin

System 2

Kidney
Foot Shao Yin

METAL

WATER

Interacts with: Foot Yang Ming Stomach
Hand Tai Yin Lung
Hand Yang Ming Large Intestine
Hand Shao Yin Heart
Hand Shao Yang Triple Warmer
Hand Tai Yang Small Intestine

Foot Tai Yin Spleen

A Reference for Interactions of Each Channel

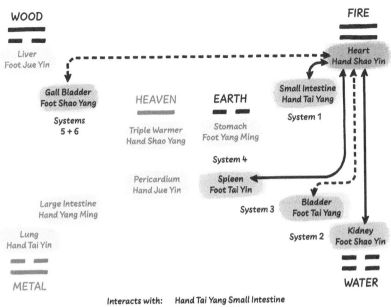

Interacts with: Hand Tai Yang Small Intestine
Foot Shao Yin Kidney
Foot Tai Yang Bladder
Foot Tai Yin Spleen
Foot Shao Yang Gall Bladder

Hand Shao Yin Heart

The Unified Acupuncture Theory

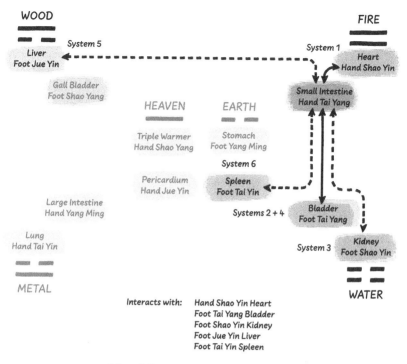

WOOD

System 5

Liver
Foot Jue Yin

Gall Bladder
Foot Shao Yang

HEAVEN

Triple Warmer
Hand Shao Yang

Pericardium
Hand Jue Yin

Large Intestine
Hand Yang Ming

Lung
Hand Tai Yin

METAL

EARTH

Stomach
Foot Yang Ming

System 6

Spleen
Foot Tai Yin

Systems 2 + 4

FIRE

System 1

Heart
Hand Shao Yin

Small Intestine
Hand Tai Yang

Bladder
Foot Tai Yang

System 3

Kidney
Foot Shao Yin

WATER

Interacts with:
Hand Shao Yin Heart
Foot Tai Yang Bladder
Foot Shao Yin Kidney
Foot Jue Yin Liver
Foot Tai Yin Spleen

Hand Tai Yang Small Intestine

A Reference for Interactions of Each Channel

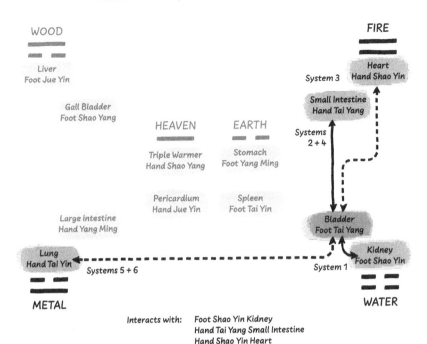

Interacts with:
Foot Shao Yin Kidney
Hand Tai Yang Small Intestine
Hand Shao Yin Heart
Hand Tai Yin Lung

Foot Tai Yang Bladder

The Unified Acupuncture Theory

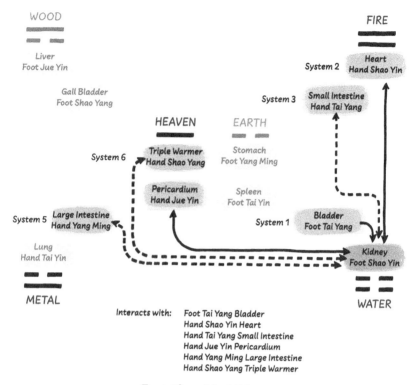

WOOD

Liver
Foot Jue Yin

Gall Bladder
Foot Shao Yang

HEAVEN

EARTH

System 6

Triple Warmer
Hand Shao Yang

Stomach
Foot Yang Ming

Pericardium
Hand Jue Yin

Spleen
Foot Tai Yin

System 5

Large Intestine
Hand Yang Ming

System 1

Bladder
Foot Tai Yang

Lung
Hand Tai Yin

METAL

FIRE

Heart
Hand Shao Yin

System 2

Small Intestine
Hand Tai Yang

System 3

Kidney
Foot Shao Yin

WATER

Interacts with: Foot Tai Yang Bladder
Hand Shao Yin Heart
Hand Tai Yang Small Intestine
Hand Jue Yin Pericardium
Hand Yang Ming Large Intestine
Hand Shao Yang Triple Warmer

Foot Shao Yin Kidney

A Reference for Interactions of Each Channel

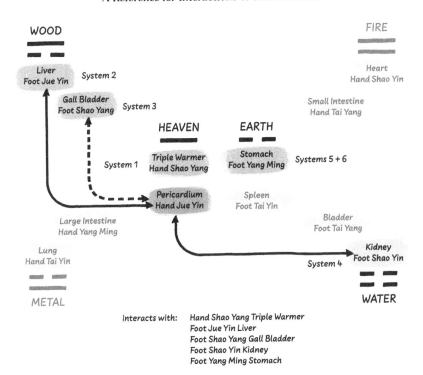

Interacts with: Hand Shao Yang Triple Warmer
Foot Jue Yin Liver
Foot Shao Yang Gall Bladder
Foot Shao Yin Kidney
Foot Yang Ming Stomach

Hand Jue Yin Pericardium

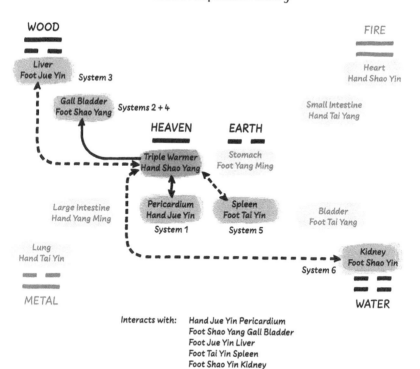

Interacts with: Hand Jue Yin Pericardium
Foot Shao Yang Gall Bladder
Foot Jue Yin Liver
Foot Tai Yin Spleen
Foot Shao Yin Kidney

Hand Shao Yang Triple Warmer

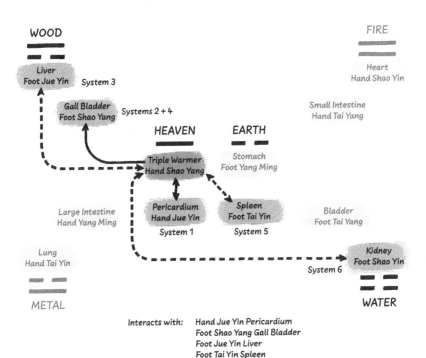

Interacts with:
Hand Jue Yin Pericardium
Foot Shao Yang Gall Bladder
Foot Jue Yin Liver
Foot Tai Yin Spleen
Foot Shao Yin Kidney

Hand Shao Yang Gall Bladder

The Unified Acupuncture Theory

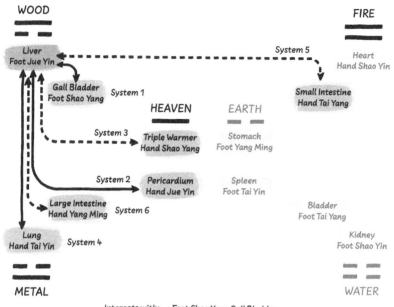

WOOD

FIRE

Liver
Foot Jue Yin

System 5

Heart
Hand Shao Yin

Gall Bladder
Foot Shao Yang

System 1

Small Intestine
Hand Tai Yang

HEAVEN

EARTH

System 3

Triple Warmer
Hand Shao Yang

Stomach
Foot Yang Ming

System 2

Pericardium
Hand Jue Yin

Spleen
Foot Tai Yin

Large Intestine
Hand Yang Ming

System 6

Bladder
Foot Tai Yang

Lung
Hand Tai Yin

System 4

Kidney
Foot Shao Yin

METAL

WATER

Interacts with: Foot Shao Yang Gall Bladder
Hand Jue Yin Pericardium
Hand Shao Yang Triple Warmer
Hand Tai Yin Lung
Hand Tai Yin Small Intestine
Hand Yang Ming Large Intestine

Foot Jue Yin Liver

HOLOGRAPHY: IMAGING AND MIRRORING

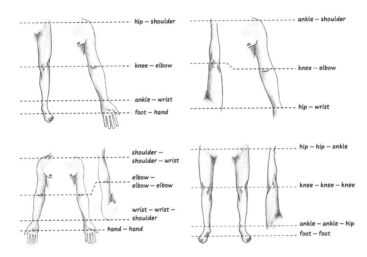

Limbs

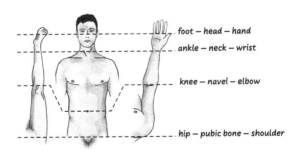

Limbs to Head and Torso

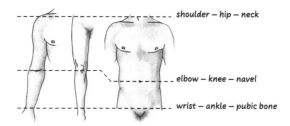

shoulder – hip – neck

elbow – knee – navel

wrist – ankle – pubic bone

Limbs to Torso

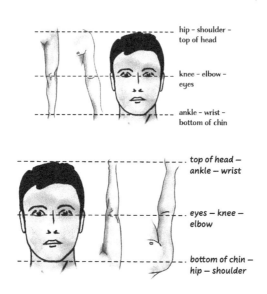

hip - shoulder -
top of head

knee - elbow -
eyes

ankle - wrist -
bottom of chin

top of head –
ankle – wrist

eyes – knee –
elbow

bottom of chin –
hip – shoulder

Limbs to Head

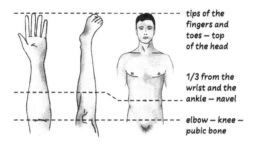

tips of the
fingers and
toes — top
of the head

1/3 from the
wrist and the
ankle — navel

elbow — knee —
pubic bone

Large Taiji

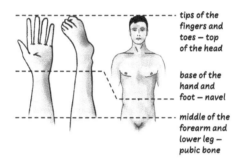

tips of the
fingers and
toes — top
of the head

base of the
hand and
foot — navel

middle of the
forearm and
lower leg —
pubic bone

Medium Taiji

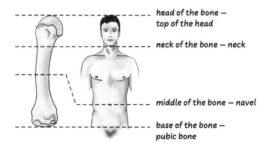

head of the bone —
top of the head

neck of the bone — neck

middle of the bone — navel

base of the bone —
pubic bone

Small Taiji